How

How to Pass Your OSCE

A Guide to Success in Nursing and Midwifery

Jacqueline Bloomfield

Anne Pegram

Carys Jones

Harlow, England • London • New York • Boston • San Francisco • Toronto
Sydney • Tokyo • Singapore • Hong Kong • Seoul • Taipei • New Delhi
Cape Town • Madrid • Mexico City • Amsterdam • Munich • Paris • Milan

Pearson Education Limited
Edinburgh Gate
Harlow
Essex CM20 2JE
England

and Associated Companies throughout the world

Visit us on the World Wide Web at:
www.pearsoned.co.uk

First published 2010

© Pearson Education Limited 2010

The rights of Jacqueline Bloomfield, Anne Pegram and Carys Jones to be identified as authors of this Work have been asserted by them in accordance with the Copyright, Designs and Patents Act 1988.

ISBN 978-0-273-72428-5

British Library Cataloguing-in-Publication Data
A catalogue record for this book is available from the British Library

Library of Congress Cataloguing-in-Publication Data
Bloomfield, Jacqueline.
  How to pass your OSCE : a guide to success in nursing and midwifery / Jacqueline Bloomfield, Anne Pegram, Carys Jones.
     p. ; cm.
  Includes bibliographical references and index.
  ISBN 978-0-273-72428-5 (pbk.)
  1. Nursing – Great Britain – Examinations – Study guides.   2. Midwifery – Great Britain – Examinations – Study guides.   I. Pegram, Anne.   II. Jones, Carys.   III. Title.
     [DNLM: 1. Education, Nursing.   2. Achievement.   3. Clinical Competence.   4. Learning.   5. Midwifery – education. WY 18 B6555h 2010]
  RT55.B56 2010
  618.2′02310076–dc22

                                                                                           2010002401

10 9 8 7 6 5 4 3 2 1
14 13 12 11 10

Typeset in 9.5/13.5pt Interstate Light by 35
Printed and bound in Great Britain by Henry Ling Ltd, Dorchester, Dorset

The publisher's policy is to use paper manufactured from sustainable forests.

Contents

Acknowledgements

The authors would like to thank the following:

- Carol Fordham-Clarke for her advice, support and expertise.
- Other colleagues with whom we work in nursing and midwifery, especially those involved in preparing students for OSCEs and examining them, and whose experiences have informed the book.
- The students who freely shared their OSCE preparation strategies and experiences with us.
- The reviewers for their valuable comments on the drafts.

Introduction

*'We don't receive wisdom, we must discover it for ourselves
after a journey that no-one can take for us or spare us.'*

MARCEL PROUST, novelist (1871-1922)

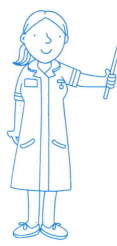

Welcome to *How to Pass Your OSCE – a guide
to success in nursing and midwifery*. We have
written this book with you in mind, to enable
you to develop a set of study skills specifically
suited to help you achieve success with your
OSCE.

Regardless of whether you are a student
or where you now are in your career as a
qualified nurse or midwife, you may be required
to undertake an Objective Structured Clinical
Examination (OSCE) as part of a course or a programme of study.
OSCEs are a valuable way of assessing proficiency in a range of
clinically-focused skills and knowledge, so they are widely used as a
fundamental assessment strategy in many programmes of nursing and
midwifery education in the United Kingdom and across the world.

For many reasons, students often find the prospect of an OSCE very
stressful. This book is not a skills textbook, nor is it a compilation of
OSCE checklists. Instead, it aims to provide nursing and midwifery
students, at all levels, with an engaging and user-friendly resource to
assist them with OSCE preparation and to help them achieve ultimate
success. We have written this book in an informal and conversational
style which we hope you will find easy to understand. We have drawn
on our extensive experience as lecturers in nursing, midwifery and
education to share with you our tips for success.

Meet the authors

Before you read any further, perhaps you might like to find out something about the authors.

Jacqueline Bloomfield

I am a registered nurse and qualified midwife and have worked in nurse education both in Australia and the UK since 2000. I am particularly interested in clinical skills and, as a lecturer, have considerable experience with OSCEs. I regularly examine OSCEs at pre- and post-qualification levels and have seen at first hand the struggles and anxiety experienced by many students in relation to this type of assessment.

Anne Pegram

Being responsible for teaching clinical skills and organising OSCEs in both pre- and post-qualification nursing, I have become increasingly aware of what helps a student to achieve success. My contribution to this book is to share my experiences of organising OSCEs as a lecturer and by using my background as a registered nurse to deconstruct the knowledge required to give an accomplished performance of the skill being examined.

Carys Jones

My areas of expertise are in language and education. I have spent many years researching how effective spoken and written communication may be achieved, particularly in multicultural environments. Over the last five years I have been involved in the development of oral and written skills in academic communication and clinical practice within nursing and midwifery studies. So my main contribution to the book is about the nature of learning and development.

Organisation of the book

This book is organised into five chapters. To set the context of the book, Chapter 1 begins by presenting background information about OSCEs. It explains what they are, and their relationship to clinical skills. In this chapter you will also learn that the OSCE provides an opportunity for students to demonstrate their ability to perform a specific clinical skill or range of skills.

In Chapter 2, you will learn about the key principles that underpin the performance and behaviour expected of you during an OSCE. This includes discussion of the importance of demonstrating the principles of infection control, documentation and record keeping, effective communication skills, maintenance of dignity and respect, and safe practice.

Chapter 3 is all about you. Entitled 'Personal learning and preparation for the OSCE', this chapter includes a series of activities to help you identify what type of learner you are and how this may affect your preparation for the OSCE.

Chapter 4 will help you with your practical preparation. Example OSCE scenarios are presented and you are given the opportunity to identify what skills and knowledge are likely to be assessed in a typical OSCE.

Chapter 5 comprises a collection of quotes and comments by students and examiners which aim to provide you with an insight into the OSCE experience. Included in this chapter are top tips for success and hints to help you avoid common pitfalls.

Throughout the book you will find a number of features to help with your learning. Quick quizzes at the end of each chapter provide opportunities to test your knowledge about what you have just learnt. Simple case studies based on realistic scenarios, reflective activities and a variety of other activities have also been included to help you to get the most out of the book. At the end of the book you will find room to write your own personalised OSCE preparation plan.

How you choose to use this book is completely up to you and will depend on your learning needs and what you hope to gain from it. You may be new to nursing or midwifery and have little idea of what an OSCE entails. In this case, understanding the common terminology will get you started; it is then recommended that you read about the basics addressed in the first few chapters before moving through the rest of the book.

For those who have previous experience of undertaking an OSCE, you may want guidance on how to maximise your potential and chances of success. If this is the case, Chapters 3 and 4 will be most relevant.

Finally, you may be pleased to have passed your OSCE but would like to be more thorough in your preparation for the next time. Reading through the whole book will help you to meet these needs.

Glossary

Let's start with the basics. Here is a glossary of terms that you will see used throughout this book.

Circuit A circuit consists of a series of activities, each of which are performed at a 'station'. Typically, a circuit has a time limit. For example, a circuit may be one hour in duration and consist of six stations.

Examiner An experienced lecturer or clinician who assesses the performance.

Killer station A station that **must** be passed in order to pass the OSCE.

KMAS An acronym used in this book to denote the four distinct components that are required when performing a clinical skill: Knowledge (K), Motor skill (M), Attitude (A) and Structure (S).

Long cases OSCEs comprising just one or two stations in which a number of skills are assessed. These may also be referred to as 'single station OSCEs'.

OSCE An acronym that stands for Objective Structured Clinical Examination.

OSCE checklist A list of the key components of the skill that the student should perform in order to demonstrate that he or she is competent, safe and thorough.

Station A position in the circuit which the student is required to visit and demonstrate a specific clinical skill, and/or the knowledge which underpins the skill within a given time limit.

Short cases OSCEs comprising a number of short stations within a circuit. These are sometimes also known as 'multi-station' OSCEs.

Patient role player An actor or service user who plays the role of the patient in a given scenario in the OSCE.

Unmanned station A station where there is no examiner present. The activity, usually in written format, is timed and requires the student to demonstrate the knowledge or theory that underpins a specific clinical skill.

Now that you know the basics, spend a few moments thinking about what you want to get from this book. Then go for it!

Jacqueline Bloomfield
Anne Pegram
Carys Jones

Chapter 1

What is an OSCE?

'Happiness comes when we test our skills towards some meaningful purpose.'

JOHN STOSSEL, Journalist (born 1947)

AIMS

At the end of this chapter, you should:

- Understand what the acronym OSCE stands for
- Understand the key features of an OSCE
- Know how OSCEs can be used to assess clinical skill competency
- Recognise the different types of OSCEs used in nursing and midwifery education

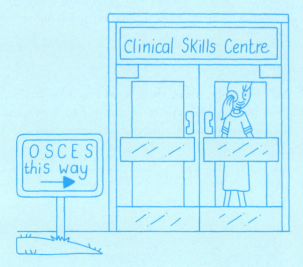

This chapter aims to equip you with the knowledge and understanding of what an OSCE is, its key features, and how it might be used to assess your competency in a range of clinical skills relevant to nursing and midwifery practice.

So what is an OSCE?

Perhaps you have just discovered that the type of assessment for the course you are studying is an OSCE. Understandably, this may have left you feeling a little apprehensive or unsure of what to expect. By the very fact that you are reading this book, you will know that the course you are studying has a clinical component. For example, it may focus on the clinical aspects integral to the provision of care for a specific patient population, such as pregnant women, or those with a particular disease, such as diabetes or asthma. Alternatively, it may be closely linked to an area of practice that requires a specific set of skills such as wound care, tissue viability or orthopaedic nursing. As such, because of the clinical focus of the course, traditional, more conventional types of assessment, such as a written exam or essay, may not be appropriate.

You may have heard other students talking about OSCEs, but perhaps you are still unclear as to what the term 'OSCE' means or what it actually involves. To answer these questions, let's start at the beginning.

ACTIVITY 1.1

Jot down some ideas about what you think an OSCE is. You may like to reflect on discussions you have had with other students or colleagues or on any information you have read about OSCEs.

....

....

....

....

....

The OSCE acronym

The term 'OSCE' is an acronym that stands for Objective Structured Clinical Examination and throughout the literature there are many different definitions. Perhaps one of the clearest is that proposed by Watson (2002, p. 424) who described the OSCE as an exam whereby 'students demonstrate their competence under a variety of simulated conditions'.

In other words, OSCEs are examinations in which the student is required to perform specific skills and behaviours in a simulated clinical or patient care environment. During an OSCE the examiner will assess your performance with regard to four distinct elements. These include the knowledge and understanding underpinning the skill (**K**); the motor or technical aspects of the skill (**M**); the affective aspects (**A**), i.e., the professional attitude associated with the performance; and structure (**S**), i.e., how you approach the skill in terms of being systematic, logical and organised. A simple acronym that can help you to remember these components is **KMAS** (Knowledge, Motor skill, Attitude, Structure). We will be discussing each of these components in greater detail later in Chapter 4.

OSCEs are not a new type of assessment. In fact, they have been used in medical education for several decades and have now become a widely accepted method of assessing clinical competence in nursing and midwifery education in the UK and in many other countries throughout the world (Rushforth 2007).

To find out more about this unique type of assessment, we will now look at each component of the OSCE acronym.

Objective (O)

'O' in the word OSCE stands for *objective* and objectivity is a defining feature of this type of assessment.

By the nature of their role, assessors have the responsibility of making professional judgements about the performance of students whom they are assessing. Within the context of nursing and midwifery, the assessor is required to make decisions based on two key judgements:

1. The extent to which a student has met the learning outcomes and standards of the particular course or subject that is being examined.

2. Whether the student has demonstrated the level of competency that is expected (Stuart 2006) and, consequently, whether the student is able to practice safely in the clinical setting.

As with all other forms of assessments, the OSCE process needs to be as transparent as possible. The OSCE is designed to achieve transparency by minimising potential bias.

But this is not as simple as it might sound. If you think for a moment about clinical practice and what you have seen while working in the practice environment, you will recognise that most practitioners have a preferred way of doing something. For example, some nurses might like to set up a sterile field in preparation for a wound dressing in a particular way, while still making sure that the key principles of asepsis are maintained. Likewise, you may have seen a colleague make a hospital bed in a slightly different way to how you or other nurses like to make it. For example, they may like to position the pillows facing away from the door while another colleague may be concerned about folding the bedspread in a specific way. Regardless of this, it is almost certain that the key principles underlying both techniques used for bedmaking are the same.

Generally, such idiosyncrasies are not problematic. However, if an examiner had a specific way of assessing student performance in accordance with her own particular likes, dislikes or habits, this could cause difficulties in terms of equity and consistency, especially if there were more than one examiner assessing the same skill. Problems would arise if students were not assessed objectively on their competence but instead on how well their performance complied with the examiner's likes and dislikes. You can see that if this were to happen, the assessment process would not be fair. In fact, it could be considered biased towards the examiner! Therefore, it is very important that the clinical exam is free from any prejudice or bias. In other words, it needs to be *objective*.

So how is this objectivity achieved in an OSCE?

Structured (S)

The letter 'S' stands for *structure*. To achieve objectivity in the assessment of competency, a clinical skill or procedure is typically broken down into component parts in a very structured way.

Imagine teaching someone how to bake a cake. Typically, you would follow a recipe and go through the various components step by step. Similarly, if you needed to teach a junior nurse or student midwife a clinical skill, it is likely that, as part of this process, you would break down the skill into its component parts. Not only would this help you to teach the skill, but it would also help the student to learn it. In fact, you may even do this without realising it.

Over to you!

ACTIVITY 1.2

Take a few minutes to reflect on how you would teach a student nurse or midwife to measure a radial pulse. Jot down some notes below.

Did your answer contain the following points?

- Explain the procedure to the student and check that they have the necessary equipment to take a radial pulse, including a watch with a second hand and an observation chart.

- Explain the importance of universal precautions and hand hygiene prior to performing any clinical skill, and ensure that the student's hands have been decontaminated.

- Explain the importance of obtaining consent from the patient prior to measuring the pulse.

- Show the student where to feel for a radial pulse on the patient's wrist, and how, by using the first and second fingers, to locate and feel the pulse.

- Demonstrate to the student how to count the number of beats for a full minute and take particular note of the rate, rhythm and strength of the pulse.

As you can see, the clinical skill of measuring a pulse has been broken down into key parts to facilitate both teaching and learning, to ensure that it is undertaken both safely and competently, and that nothing is missed.

When planning for the OSCE, a team of course lecturers will spend time considering in detail each of the skills that will be examined. Each skill will be broken down into its component parts, and marking criteria, in the form of a checklist, will be developed. Essentially, this is a list of the key components of the skill that the student should perform in order to demonstrate that he is competent, safe and thorough. For example, in the following excerpt from a marking checklist, the key components inherent to the skill of feeding a dependent patient have been identified.

1	Decontaminates hands before starting the procedure, using the recommended technique.
2	Dons an apron to protect clothing and prevent cross-infection.
3	Explains the procedure to the patient and gains their consent.
4	Ensures that the patient is positioned comfortably and is ready for their meal.
5	Protects the patient's clothing from spillages with a clean towel or apron.
6	Explains to the patient what is on the plate and asks about their food preferences.

During the examination the assessor will use the checklist to mark each student's performance. This is typically done by observing if each part of the skill has been performed and whether it has been demonstrated correctly and safely. By using such a structured approach any examiner bias is substantially minimised as they can only mark a student's performance in accordance with whether the student has or has not met each criterion set out on the marking sheet. The allocation of marks between different stations will be agreed upon by the examiners in advance of the OSCE and the student's final score will usually be based on the overall number of correct responses on the marking criteria checklist, as shown in this example:

Feeding a dependent patient	Yes	No	Score
1 Decontaminates hands before starting the procedure, using the recommended technique.	✔		1
2 Dons an apron to protect clothing and prevent cross-infection.		✔	0
3 Explains the procedure to the patient and gains their consent.	✔		1
4 Ensures that the patient is positioned comfortably and is ready for their meal.	✔		1
5 Protects the patient's clothing from spillages with a clean towel or apron.		✔	0
6 Explains to the patient what is on the plate and asks about their food preferences.	✔		1

Another way in which OSCEs can be considered to be a structured form of assessment is the way in which they are organised. OSCEs consist of different types of assessment tasks, which will be considered later in this chapter. For now, we will consider the most typical OSCEs, which consist of a circuit or series of short activities, each of which must be performed at a different 'station'. These activities are timed and students are assessed at each station by one examiner using the predetermined, objective marking sheet. In this way, each student is assessed in both a structured and standardised way, thereby eliminating the risk of inequality and inconsistency. By now, you will be starting to get an idea of what OSCEs are all about; but there is more. Read on.

Clinical (C)

By their very nature OSCEs are *clinically* focused assessments: hence the third letter 'C' in the OSCE acronym. You may know from experience that a typical clinical environment is often busy with multidisciplinary team members working to meet the needs of the numerous patients or clients for whom they are caring. Sometimes, when performing a clinical skill in the practice setting, it is not unusual to be interrupted or distracted by what else is happening. But clinical skills are fundamental to nursing and midwifery practice, and specific skills are often needed for patients who are very ill, experiencing pain or who are emotionally distressed. Therefore, in many cases it would be inappropriate or even unethical for an examination to be conducted in the clinical setting or for a skill to be demonstrated several times by many different students using a real patient. Likewise, it would be unrealistic to expect a patient to recount his history repeatedly for the purpose of an OSCE.

To overcome these issues, simulation is commonly used for OSCEs in order to create an environment similar to that of the clinical setting. A variety of approaches can be used. Some examples include:

- A simple model of the skin can be used to enable the student to demonstrate how to give an intramuscular injection.

- Sophisticated manikins can be programmed to mimic a rapidly deteriorating patient on whom the student can be required to demonstrate a range of skills.

- Professional actors or service users can take on the role of a patient to enable students to perform a certain skill, such as measuring a radial pulse or history-taking, which involves demonstrating effective communication.

To set the scene at the beginning of each station, the student will be given a short scenario to read. This will provide the information necessary to establish the context in which the specific set of skills is to be performed and will identify the skills being examined.

Now, over to you again!

ACTIVITY 1.3

Consider the following examples. Can you identify which skills are being assessed? Jot down your answers in the space provided.

Example 1

You are asked to assist Mr Okara with his midday meal. Demonstrate the procedure you would use to wash your hands before commencing this task.

Skill being assessed ....

Example 2

Mrs Green is Day 1 post-elective caesarean section. You are required to undertake a post-partum assessment. Undertake this procedure and document your findings.

Skills being assessed ....

Example 3

Mrs Lee has presented to Accident and Emergency with a painful right shoulder which she reports injuring while playing tennis earlier today. Undertake an appropriate nursing history including pain assessment.

Skills being assessed ....

You will find the answers at the end of the book.

Examination (E)

The final letter in the OSCE acronym stands for *examination*. An examination is the process of testing competence or knowledge. As such, in an OSCE, clinical competency is assessed by breaking it down into its various components. In this way students are required to demonstrate not only *what they know* but also that they *know how* to perform a clinical skill. Therefore, they must also *show how* to perform it competently by demonstrating the necessary *actions* required for the execution of the skill in a safe, appropriate and competent manner.

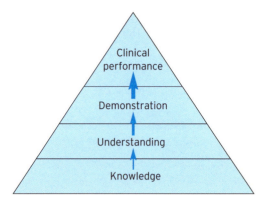

Figure 1.1 From acquiring knowledge to applying knowledge
Source: Adapted from Miller 1990, p. S63.

Miller recommends that, in order to demonstrate competency, 'knows', 'knows how', 'shows how' and 'does' (Miller 1990, p. S63) are necessary. This means that, in terms of demonstrating clinical competency, knowledge (knows), competence (knows how), demonstration (shows how) and clinical performance (does) are all important, as illustrated in Figure 1.1.

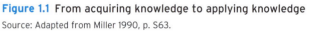

Knowing, showing, doing

To illustrate the above, let's look at the example of pain assessment, which is a skill that is fundamental to both nursing and midwifery practice. If, as part of an OSCE, you were required to undertake a pain assessment on a simulated patient/client, the examiner would assess you on the following clinical competences:

Knowledge

This is at the bottom of the triangle, indicating that it is the most basic and broadest component in the framework. It relates to having the appropriate knowledge that underpins practice. Pain is a very complex phenomenon. Because of this, adequate knowledge and understanding of the potential physiological, psychological and emotional elements of pain is required in order to effectively undertake a pain assessment. Knowledge and understanding of the different types of pain and how these may relate to an individual is also important.

Understanding

This is a higher component in the framework because it depends on *knowing how* to do something and *understanding why* it should be done in a certain way. In the given example, this would involve demonstrating knowledge and understanding of how pain assessment can be effectively undertaken, including the use of appropriate communication skills. Knowledge of different pain assessment tools and how to use them is important. Likewise, knowing how to interpret data obtained from a pain assessment is also essential.

Demonstration

This is a further step up in the framework because it depends on demonstrating or *showing how* to do something. It requires familiarity with the process of pain assessment and with demonstrating how to perform the assessment in a systematic and structured way.

Clinical performance

The performance or the 'doing' part is the most important and, sometimes, most challenging part. It requires integrating all three previous points and performing the skill in a professionally competent way. In this example, it includes communicating with the patient, assessing her pain using an appropriate method, documenting it and interpreting the findings.

Now what?

You may wonder how the triangle depicted in Figure 1.1 fits with the OSCE. This is a very good question. Read on.

If we reconsider the key requirements of an OSCE you will recall that they need to be objective and structured. To meet these requirements the OSCE is conducted in a simulated environment and all students are assessed in the same way, by examiners using a structured checklist. It is also important that any actors playing the role of a patient behave in a consistent manner. This will help to maximise standardisation and consistency of the examination.

For example, if a patient interview scenario was being used to assess communication skills, it would be important that the patient role player communicates the same information to each student. Likewise, if an actor/patient role player's pulse rate was being measured as part of an OSCE station, it is important that this is stable and free from any significant fluctuations that might compromise standardisation. In practice, such standardisation is not possible, as every patient and client is different. Furthermore, the environments in which they are cared for are also very different. For example, there are many variables that may influence pulse rate. The 'does', identified in Miller's model, relates to the ability to integrate knowledge and practice, and to adapt this to the needs of individual patients and clients. The OSCE provides an opportunity for an assessment of competency within in a simulated environment. However, the 'doing' part requires this competency to be demonstrated in practice.

So far, we have looked at the OSCE in general, as a good way of assessing clinical skills. But the OSCE involves more than this. Read on.

Types of OSCEs

Now that you know what an OSCE is, the next part of this chapter will consider different types of OSCEs and the context in which these may be used within nursing and midwifery education. It is important to recognise that different universities may manage and deliver *OSCEs* differently. However, there are two main types of OSCEs:

1. OSCEs comprising a number of short stations within a circuit

These are known as 'short cases' or 'multi-station OSCEs' and are typically used to assess pre-registration students. For example, the OSCE may last an hour, during which time students rotate around six stations, demonstrating a simple clinical skill at each station. In this case each station would be 10 minutes' duration. In addition to skills, some OSCEs may also comprise knowledge stations.

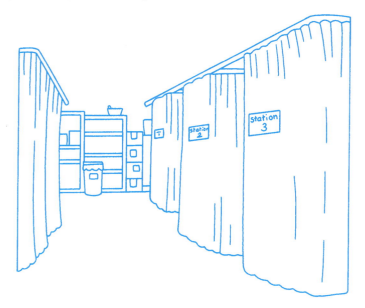

2. OSCEs comprising just one or two stations in which a number of skills are assessed

These are usually referred to as 'long cases' or 'single stations' and are most commonly used for post-qualification students or students nearing the end of their pre-registration programmes. They are typically used to assess competency in the integration of skills. This type of OSCE may be one hour long, but comprise just one station, lasting the whole hour, or two stations, each one of 30 minutes' duration. As part of a 'long case', knowledge may be tested while a procedure is undertaken or after the skills component has been completed. For example, this may involve the examiner asking questions about what has been done and why.

It is also useful to recognise that some OSCEs may include what is known as an 'unmanned station'. This type of station typically involves an activity, usually in written format, that requires the student to demonstrate the knowledge or theory that underpins a specific clinical skill. Although timed, there will be no examiner present at the station.

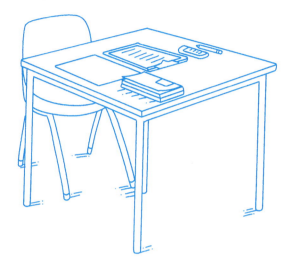

Why do OSCEs differ?

You might be wondering why there are different models of OSCEs and why OSCEs differ in length. These are important considerations. The difference in length will commonly reflect the stage a student or practitioner has reached in her programme of nursing or midwifery studies. For example, it would be appropriate to expect an OSCE for an experienced midwife studying at Masters level to be more complex than one undertaken by first-year student nurses studying at under-graduate level. Let's consider two more examples.

Example 1

You are a pre-registration nursing student approaching the end of your first year. You have discovered that you will have an OSCE to assess your clinical skills in the course that you have been taking. In this course you have studied the skills clusters required by the Nursing and Midwifery Council (NMC) regulations (NMC 2007) and subsequently learnt a number of clinical skills that are fundamental to nursing practice.

It is likely that the OSCE for this student would focus on the assessment of competence in a range of fundamental skills taught and, above all, the student would be required to demonstrate knowledge of key principles, safety and accuracy. In this type of OSCE the stations would be developed with a focus on discrete skills, such as aseptic technique, hand decontamination or measurement of vital signs, rather than on the more complex integration of skills.

Example 2

You are an experienced post-qualification midwife undertaking a Masters course in sexual health. The clinical component of the course requires you to demonstrate competency in skills related to cervical screening, health promotion and family planning.

It is likely that the OSCE for this course would focus on assessing competence in the skills learnt, but you would also be expected to demonstrate the integration of those skills. For example, you would need to demonstrate not only how to perform the cervical screening procedure but also competency in the provision of health education, family planning and the ability to effectively answer any questions that the client in the scenario may ask.

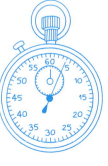

In other words, the OSCE is designed to assess competency in skills that are fundamental to nursing practice and to do so at different levels of complexity, depending on what stage you have reached in the programme. The first OSCE is to assess how you perform the basic skills required for a range of different tasks while later OSCEs assess how well you are able to integrate appropriate skills in specific patient scenarios.

Recap and recall

You have reached the end of this chapter and you should now have a sound understanding of what OSCEs are. To check your understanding of the key points we have covered, spend some time asking yourself the following questions:

- Do I know what the acronym OSCE stands for?
- Do I understand the key features of an OSCE?
- Do I know how OSCEs can be used to assess clinical skill competency?
- Can I recognise different types of OSCEs including long and short cases?

Quick quiz

You might also like to test your knowledge and understanding with this quick quiz. You will find the correct answers at the end of the book.

Multiple choice

Choose the best answer from the options provided.

1. A key feature on an Objective Structured Clinical Examination is:

   A. Subjectivity
   B. Objectivity
   C. Variability
   D. Flexibility

2. The letter 'C' in the OSCE acronym stands for which of the following?

   A. Complex
   B. Clarity
   C. Credible
   D. Clinical

3. Typically, OSCEs comprise a circuit containing a number of:

   A. Stations
   B. Assessments
   C. Actors
   D. Examiners

4. Which of the following is primarily used by an examiner during an OSCE to assess a student's performance?

   A. A written essay
   B. A structured checklist
   C. Actor feedback
   D. Student feedback

True or false

Identify whether the following statements are true or false.

5. An OSCE is typically used in nursing and midwifery to assess skill competency.

   True ☐   False ☐

6. OSCEs are new types of assessment used exclusively in nursing and midwifery education.

   True ☐   False ☐

Chapter 2

Essential principles underpinning OSCEs

'Back of every noble life there are principles that have fashioned it.'

GEORGE HORACE LORIMER, Publisher (1867-1937)

AIMS

At the end of this chapter you should:

- Understand the key principles that govern nursing and midwifery practice
- Recognise how these key principles may be assessed during an OSCE
- Know what behaviour is expected during an OSCE in terms of etiquette and professional behaviour

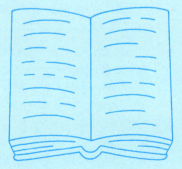

Essential principles underpinning performance and behaviour

In this chapter consideration is given to the key principles that underpin performance and behaviour during an OSCE. These are no different to those that govern professional practice for a registered nurse or midwife or those that are required by student health professionals. They are essential for upholding professional standards and ensuring the provision of safe, quality patient care.

ACTIVITY 2.1

Before moving on, spend a few minutes considering which professional guidelines and policy underpin clinical practice in relation to patient care delivery. Make a list of any that you can think of below.

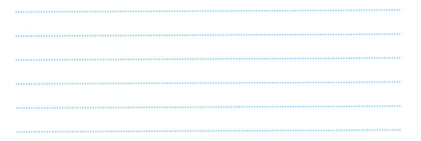

How did you do? It is likely that you have come across many different policies and guidelines while in practice. Perhaps your list included things such as:

- The Code: Standards of conduct, performance and ethics for nurses and midwives (NMC 2008a)

- National and local policies including:
  - Standards for medicines management (NMC 2008b)
  - Midwives rules and standards (NMC 2004)
  - Guidance for the care of older people (NMC 2009)
  - Evidence-based practice in infection control (NICE 2003)
  - National hand-washing campaign guidelines (RCN 2005)
  - The NHS Knowledge and Skills Framework (DoH 2004)

- Risk assessment tools and guidance such as the Waterlow risk assessment tool
- Essence of Care benchmarks (DoH 2001, 2003, 2007)
- University guidelines such as those contained in a Practice Placement handbook relevant to your programme or place of study.

Although there are many more professional guidelines, from this list core principles of practice can be identified, and these are essential for safe practice in meeting the care needs of patients and clients. These principles are:

- infection control
- safe practice
- accurate documentation and record-keeping
- effective communication
- maintenance of dignity and respect.

Because these principles are so important when performing clinical skills in the practice environment, each one could be examined separately during an OSCE. Alternatively, the examiner may be looking for knowledge and demonstration of these principles incorporated in a set of skills required to be performed.

In this chapter you will have the opportunity to explore how these principles might relate to a specific OSCE scenario. Let's now consider each one in turn.

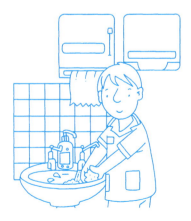

1. Infection control

Hospital-acquired infections are a considerable problem in practice and it is imperative that all health professionals are skilled in the practice of infection control.

ACTIVITY 2.2

Before moving on, spend a few minutes considering what the term 'standard precautions' means and how this works in practice. Jot down a few ideas below.

How did you do? Compare your ideas with the following definition.

> 'Standard precautions, also referred to as universal precautions, are simple infection control measures that reduce the risk of transmission of blood-borne pathogens through exposure to blood or body fluids among patients and healthcare workers.'   (WHO 2005)

> 'Standard precautions incorporate nine elements of practice aimed at preventing or minimising the risk of cross-infection.'   (ICNA 2003)

These precautions include:

- hand hygiene
- personal protective equipment (PPE)
- safe use and disposal of sharps
- safe handling and disposal of waste
- safe management of laundry
- decontamination of equipment
- maintenance of a clean environment
- personal hygiene
- food hygiene.

As you will appreciate, it is essential that the guidelines surrounding standard precautions are rigorously followed by all healthcare workers due to the risk of exposure to blood, body fluids and other infectious agents.

2. Safe practice

Ways in which safe practice can be demonstrated during the OSCE will very much be determined by the specific scenario. However, you will not be required to perform any tasks that are beyond the scope of your practice in terms of what you have been taught. Always remember that, in an OSCE, safe practice will primarily be concerned with the environment in which you work and the equipment that you may use.

Maintaining a safe environment is essential and, within any health-care environment, risk assessments should be undertaken before engaging in care activities or performing clinical skills. Take a moment to reflect on your own experiences in practice and consider some of the risk assessments that you regularly undertake in practice.

Some examples of commonly used risk assessments include those related to moving and handling patients, slips, trips and falls, swallowing ability, skin assessment and checking equipment before it is used.

Inspecting the environment for potential hazards such as spills or obstacles which might be dangerous is also important, and, although it is unlikely that you will encounter these things in the context of an OSCE station, the examiner will expect you to show an awareness of key safety issues.

Ensuring that equipment is in working order and is used correctly is also vital to maintain the safety and comfort of patients and for accuracy of results and any assessments that may be undertaken.

3. Accurate documentation and record-keeping

The importance of accurate and timely documentation cannot be underestimated, as stipulated in the relevant NMC guidelines (NMC 2007). Many OSCE scenarios will require documentation following the completion of a patient assessment or procedure. For example, ensuring that a signature clearly indicates that medication has been administered may form part of an OSCE.

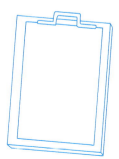

Documentation and record-keeping are an important part of the OSCE because they show not only how well you can perform this task but also your understanding of the key principles underpinning effective written communication. These include things such as the appropriate use of terminology and precise language, objectivity, timeliness, attention to legibility, and accuracy of information.

ACTIVITY 2.3

Examine the observation chart (Figure 2.1): comment on the quality of documentation with regard to legibility and accuracy, and identify any omissions.

Use the space below to make your comments.

....

....

....

....

....

....

When you are ready, check your answers with those at the end of the book.

4. Effective communication

As previously discussed, any one or more of the core principles could be examined on their own in an OSCE and this includes communication skills. Demonstrating an understanding of the principles of what constitutes effective verbal and non-verbal communication is essential, especially if an actor playing a patient role is included in any of the tasks because how you interact with that person will also be noted.

At this point, you might spend a few minutes thinking about the kinds of verbal and non-verbal communication skills that will be expected of a nurse or midwife when caring for a patient in a practice setting. In order to think about them, let's start with the basic point: communication has to be effective for the best interests of the patient to be served. So the following question needs to answered: In what ways can communication between a nurse or midwife and the patient that they are caring for be effective?

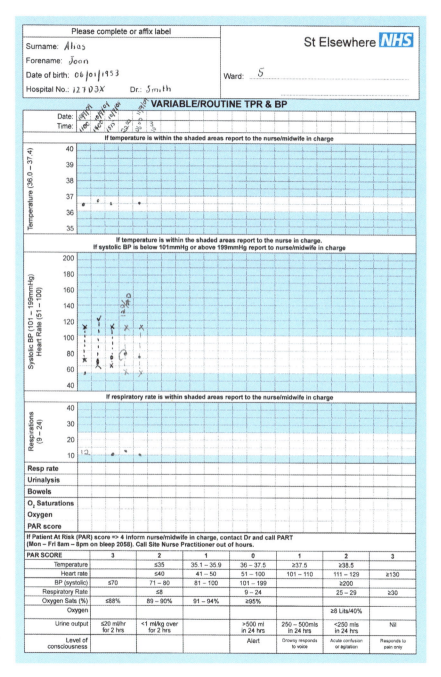

Figure 2.1 Observation chart

ACTIVITY 2.4

Spend a few minutes writing down some ideas before you read on.

....

....

....

....

....

....

You may have thought of the following:

> The patient needs to feel valued, comfortable about the communication, able to talk freely and trust the nurse or midwife with whom she is communicating. The patient also needs to know that what he is saying is being heard and the likely implications of the communication.

Now think of the verbal and non-verbal communication skills that are most likely to promote effective communication. Jot a few notes below before you read on.

....

....

....

....

....

....

Perhaps you identified a combination of verbal and non-verbal skills. For example:

Verbal	Non-verbal
Using open questions	Making eye contact
Asking one question at a time, not several questions, and following up	Showing active listening
Paraphrasing and seeking clarification to check understanding	Showing sensitive body language such as an open posture

Such skills of communication should always be evident whenever you are caring for a patient or client and whenever you are communicating with their family or friends or with any other health professional. Therefore, you will be expected to demonstrate them during the OSCE.

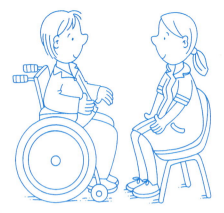

In addition to knowing what comprises effective communication, it is also crucial that you show an understanding of why these skills are important. For example:

- Open questions promote conversation and trust.
- Eye contact shows interest.
- Being listened to makes a patient feel valued.
- An open posture will encourage a patient to ask questions.

Demonstrating these attributes is essential during an OSCE because, like a real patient, a role player would like to feel that you are genuinely interested in her and not just performing a series of tasks in an impersonal and mechanical manner as if you have a checklist to complete.

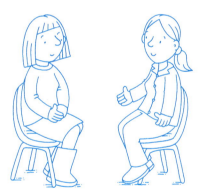

Also, don't forget: You will need to show that you are communicating effectively and appropriately with the examiner.

5. Maintenance of dignity and respect

A number of recent professional directives and government recommendations have reinforced the importance of treating all patients with dignity and respect (DoH 2001, 2003, 2007). So you will also be required to demonstrate these values throughout the OSCE process. Dignity and respect are essential professional values. In the OSCE they must be evident in your interactions with the role player, the examiners and your student colleagues.

By being present at the OSCE, the actor will have consented to being involved in a patient role, so it is essential that professional values are upheld throughout the simulated interaction. Showing dignity and respect will involve obtaining consent, checking the role player's preferences in terms of how they wish to be addressed, protecting modesty and privacy, and communicating in a respectful and courteous way.

As discussed in Chapter 1, because an OSCE is a formal examination, you will also be expected to show respect towards the examiners and your student colleagues. Ways in which this can be done include by following instructions, not disrupting other students during the examination, and communicating in an appropriate manner.

Now, over to you!

Putting it into practice

We have now addressed the essential principles underpinning nursing and midwifery care that will be examined in an OSCE. Let's apply these principles to a typical OSCE scenario.

ACTIVITY 2.5

Consider the following scenario. You are caring for Alice, a patient with intravenous (IV) therapy. You are required to assess her cannula site and to document your findings on the chart below.

Intravenous cannula site assessment record			
Date and time of assessment	Yes	No	Comments
Check date of insertion of cannula			
Assess IV dressing is intact			
Assess IV access site for swelling			
Assess IV access site for redness			
Assess IV access site for tracking			
Assess IV access site for leaking			
Name, signature and designation			

Identify how you could demonstrate knowledge and practice of each of the five essential principles underpinning nursing and midwifery care. Remember that these are:

- infection control
- safe practice
- accurate documentation and record-keeping
- effective communication
- maintenance of dignity and respect.

Jot down some notes below.

....

....

....

....

....

....

Here are some examples that you could have identified in relation to principles of good practice.

Infection control

Hand decontamination should be performed at both the beginning and the end of the assessment procedure. Standard precautions should also be demonstrated including the appropriate use of an apron and gloves.

Safe practice

Demonstrating safe practice would require you to check the environment before taking any further action in the assessment procedure. This would include:

- checking that the height of the bed is appropriate to avoid unnecessary back strain;
- taking note of when the patient's cannula was inserted and when it is due to be changed.

As you will know, these checks are an integral part of the assessment process.

Accurate documentation and record-keeping

The date and time of the assessment should be noted on the assessment chart. Additionally, your writing must be legible and any descriptive language should be relevant to the type of assessment undertaken. Your signature and designation will clearly identify who has undertaken the assessment.

Effective communication

In addition to the above points, suitable language should be used to explain the procedure and findings to the actor playing the role of the patient. This will incorporate using appropriate tone, volume, pitch and intonation in your speech, and demonstrating effective non-verbal skills, in terms of body language.

Maintenance of dignity and respect

Consent should be obtained from the actor/patient prior to performing the skill. The dignity of the role player should be maintained by limiting any unnecessary exposure.

It is important to ensure that all aspects of professional practice are included in your repertoire of essential skills. At OSCEs, too, they are considered to be an essential component of patient care. Even if they are not the direct focus of assessment, they will be assessed indirectly.

Recap and recall

You have now reached the end of Chapter 2 and you should have a sound understanding of the essential principles underpinning OSCEs. To check your understanding of the key points that we have covered, spend some time asking yourself the following questions:

- Do I understand the key principles that govern nursing and midwifery practice?

- Can I recognise how these key principles may be assessed during an OSCE?

- Do I know what behaviour is expected from me during an OSCE in terms of etiquette and professional behaviour?

Quick quiz

You might also like to test your knowledge and understanding with this quick quiz. You will find the correct answers at the end of the book.

Multiple choice

Choose the best answer from the options provided.

1. Simple measures used to reduce the transmission of infection are commonly referred to as:

   A. Standard or universal precautions
   B. Global precautions
   C. Hygiene standards
   D. Infection protection

2. Undertaking a risk assessment is an essential requirement for which of the following?

   A. Effective communication
   B. Safe practice
   C. Maintaining dignity and respect
   D. Maintaining staff and patient satisfaction

3. A relevant way of demonstrating dignity and respect towards a patient/patient actor during an OSCE is:

   A. Ignoring them during the examination
   B. Asking how they would like to be addressed
   C. Telling them what you would like to be called
   D. Introducing yourself to the examiner

4. Which of the following is an example of non-verbal communication?

    A. An open-ended question

    B. Paraphrasing what has been said

    C. Speaking clearly and loudly

    D. Making eye contact

True or false

Identify whether the following statements are true or false.

5. Effective communication underpins the safe and effective care of all patients and clients.

    True ❑   False ❑

6. During an OSCE, students are expected to behave in a professional way.

    True ❑   False ❑

Chapter 3

Personal learning and preparation for the OSCE

'The mind can only see what it is prepared to see.'

DR EDWARD DE BONO, Leading authority in creative thinking (born 1933)

AIMS

By the end of this chapter, you should know:

- Why preparing for the OSCE is important
- How to be an effective learner
- Why being an effective learner is important for the OSCE

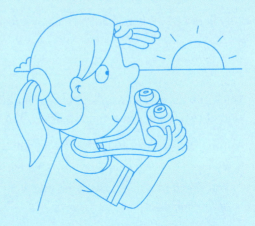

After working through the first two chapters, you probably have a good idea about what the OSCE is like and the standards of nursing practice that you need to be successful.

This chapter is about you and the way you learn in relation to preparing for the OSCE. Understanding what the OSCE is like is only a part of what you need to think about in advance. The other, much bigger, part is to do with knowing yourself as a student. Do you learn effectively? The quality of your learning is important because it will underpin your performance in the exam.

As you read through this chapter and do the activities, you may find that there is much more to being an effective learner than you realised. So try not to race through the chapter too speedily. Take time to think about the ideas so that you can internalise them gradually.

Being an effective learner

So what is an effective learner? Or, more to the point – how effective a learner are you? Or perhaps – how effective a learner can you become? As you read on, you should find the way of learning that suits you best as you prepare for the OSCE.

ACTIVITY 3.1

Spend a few minutes thinking about the four questions below and keep them at the back of your mind as you work through this chapter.

Why is the OSCE important? Think of a few reasons.

....

....

Think about yourself as a student preparing to take the OSCE. What kind of result are you aiming to achieve: A, B or C?

A. You want to excel and achieve the highest grade possible. ❏

B. You would like to gain a comfortable pass. ❏

C. You would be satisfied with the minimum grade to get a
   borderline pass. ❏

Thinking about the OSCE, what do you do well and what do you need to work on?

....

....

How are you likely to approach the OSCE? Tick the appropriate box to indicate how far you agree or disagree with the following statements. (1 = completely disagree, 4 = completely agree)

	1	2	3	4
A. You feel that your first experience of the OSCE is going to be a test case for finding out how you react to it and how well you perform.	❏	❏	❏	❏
B. You think that your best strategy is to ask other students who have experienced the OSCE for their perceptions of what it is like.	❏	❏	❏	❏
C. You feel that you should follow the advice given to you by the lecturers who run the OSCE.	❏	❏	❏	❏
D. You feel that you need to find out as much as you can about the exam from your lecturers and other students.	❏	❏	❏	❏
E. You feel that you need to understand the purpose of the OSCE before you set about preparing for it.	❏	❏	❏	❏
F. You feel that you understand the purpose of the OSCE and that you can pass it.	❏	❏	❏	❏
G. You feel that you understand the purpose of the OSCE and you need time to prepare for it.	❏	❏	❏	❏

Your responses to these statements will suggest to you what type of learner you are, especially if you read on.

Why and how do we learn?

Let's deal with 'why' first. What do you think? What motivates you to learn? Think about this in relation to the OSCE and jot down some ideas below.

....

....

....

....

....

....

Now read on.

You may be motivated to learn in order to pass the OSCE, which is a necessary requirement for your professional development. This is known as *extrinsic* motivation. On the other hand, you may be motivated to learn because you are interested in and enthusiastic about the subject as a whole. This is known as *intrinsic* motivation.

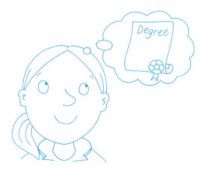

Both types of motivation are important for passing an exam. Being extrinsically motivated may be very helpful for achieving a good result but intrinsic motivation is much better and much safer because it means thinking about how and why exams are an essential part of professional development. So you will want to think beyond the OSCE. You will not see it simply as an exam that has to be passed so that you can qualify, but more as a vehicle that enables you to enhance your knowledge and understanding as far as possible.

If your learning is driven by extrinsic motivation, you may be losing out without realising it. Even if you find the OSCE easy to prepare for, you are likely to think of it as an end in itself – something you have to pass regardless of whether or not the experience of preparing for it is worthwhile. But you could think of it as being something much more effective in the long term. You could think of it as a means of preparing yourself for further challenges as you progress from one level to another. Then the learning process becomes personally much more enriching and rewarding than it would be if you were only interested in getting through each exam. In other words, become a life-long learner.

Now let's consider the second part of the question 'How'.

This is the really important part. So, how do you learn? Again, in relation to the OSCE, think about this for a few minutes and jot down a few ideas below.

....

....

....

....

....

....

Now let's think about two types of learners: 'surface' and 'deep' (Entwistle 1997). Perhaps you can guess what the difference is between them. Which type of learner do you think you are?

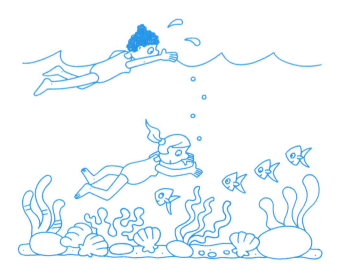

ACTIVITY 3.2

Decide which of the following items describe a surface learner and which describe a deep learner. Tick the appropriate box.

Learning behaviour	Surface	Deep
Intending to cope with the course requirements	❑	❑
Intending to understand ideas for oneself	❑	❑
Treating the course as unrelated bits of knowledge	❑	❑
Relating ideas to previous knowledge and experience	❑	❑
Looking for patterns and underlying principles	❑	❑
Memorising facts and procedures routinely	❑	❑

(adapted from Entwistle 1997, p. 19)

You can check your answers at the end of the book.

You may have realised two things about a deep approach to learning. First, it is much more effective than a surface approach. Second, it is likely to be underpinned by intrinsic, not extrinsic, motivation.

So, be careful! If you think you might be a surface learner, you may find yourself becoming unnecessarily pressurised and worried about your studies and the OSCE. But if you are a deep learner, you will be actively interested in your course and able to fully appreciate what the OSCE is all about.

For a deep approach to be really effective, it is important to develop good learning strategies (Entwistle and McCune 2004).

Being strategic

Becoming a good strategic learner
helps you not only to prepare for
the OSCE, but to understand the
essence of nursing as a caring
profession and to be a health
professional who is both well-
informed and caring.

Now for your ideas!

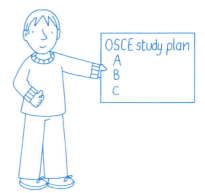

ACTIVITY 3.3

Think of some good learning strategies and jot them down below.

....

....

....

....

....

....

Do any of your ideas fit into the following broad descriptions sug-
gested by Entwistle (1997, p. 19)?

- 'aiming to achieve the highest possible grades'
- 'putting consistent effort into studying'
- 'finding the right conditions and materials for studying'
- 'managing time and effort effectively'.

Let's think about each one separately.

'Aiming to achieve the highest possible grades'

Notice that this is not just about aiming to pass, but aiming high. Why
is this important? Well, it not only means you have a better chance of

passing, but you are likely to think deeply about what the OSCE is set up to test and why.

'Putting consistent effort into studying'

This may seem an obvious strategy. But perhaps it is worth remembering that effective studying really does need 'consistent effort'. Developing your brain through thinking about and questioning new knowledge as you study helps you to deepen your understanding of new facts, concepts and ways of doing things.

'Finding the right conditions and materials for studying'

This is about you personally and your unique way of working. The 'conditions and materials' that suit one student do not necessarily suit another. We all have to find our best ways of studying that make us feel most comfortable and confident. The 'finding' may take time and effort but – don't give up, be persistent – developing this strategy is very important.

'Managing time and effort effectively'

You may be able to appreciate how this strategy overlaps with the other three. Time management is fundamental to any effective studying. By being well organised you are giving yourself the best chance both to be successful in everything you do and to develop professionally.

Looking for cues

As you prepare for the OSCE one good strategy is to look for cues: cues about what to expect, what is going to be assessed, and how it is going to be assessed. Some students are better than others at doing this. Students tend to fall into three types: the cue-deaf, the cue-conscious and the cue-seeking (Rowntree 1988, pp. 45–46).

So how do different students prepare? Your turn now!

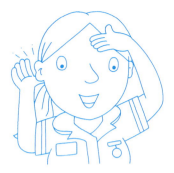

ACTIVITY 3.4

Read the descriptions of Student A, Student B and Student C described below. Are they cue-deaf, cue-conscious or cue-seeking?

Student A

Student A believes that she should watch out for cues that might be useful to her in the exam. She thinks that staff might drop hints about which kinds of things are likely or unlikely to come up in the OSCE. Although it could be a matter of luck, she hopes this strategy will help her to pass.

Student B

Student B actively watches out for cues by having as much interaction with the staff as possible. He deliberately asks relevant and thoughtful questions and refers to examples from his experiences and his reading. He also tries to catch a tutor alone and encourage some chatting about the OSCE.

Student C

Student C believes it would be too risky to rely on guesswork and on staff dropping hints about which subjects or questions will come up. She thinks that the only way to prepare for the OSCE is to work as hard as she can.

Write down your answers, and reasons, below.

Student A: ....

....

Student B: ....

....

Student C: ....

....

All three students are strategic in their own ways. They are thinking about the OSCE well in advance: about the kinds of knowledge they need and how to prepare. Perhaps the most active student is Student B, who is 'seeking cues'. Student A is also fairly active because she is 'cue-conscious'. Student C is definitely 'cue-deaf'. Although she is probably a very conscientious worker, she may not be managing her efforts as well as she might. She has set herself a plan that she can work with independently but she might be rather isolated.

So what kind of learner are you?

ACTIVITY 3.5

Think about the following questions in turn and tick the appropriate box.

	A	B	C
When introduced to some important new information, do you:			
A. Like to approach it with a blank sheet?	❑	❑	❑
B. Feel you need to link it to your prior knowledge in some way?	❑	❑	❑
C. Feel uncertain about how you will react?	❑	❑	❑
When something is explained to you, do you:			
A. Need to accept that explanation, word for word?	❑	❑	❑
B. Feel you need to link it to your prior knowledge in some way?	❑	❑	❑
C. Not know how you will react?	❑	❑	❑
When learning about something new, do you:			
A. Like to ask questions straight away?	❑	❑	❑
B. Like to go away and think about it first and then ask questions?	❑	❑	❑
C. Prefer to accept what you have been told?	❑	❑	❑

A   B   C

How do you react to new challenges? Are you likely to:

A. Become stressed and anxious? ☐ ☐ ☐

B. Enjoy it? ☐ ☐ ☐

C. Become stressed, but enjoy it? ☐ ☐ ☐

Do you think assessment and learning:

A. Are not related? ☐ ☐ ☐

B. Are related? ☐ ☐ ☐

C. May be related? ☐ ☐ ☐

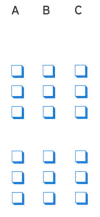

If you ticked most of the A boxes, you may not be thinking deeply enough about what you are doing. If you feel that you need to experience situations in order to learn, your level of learning will be superficial because you will not have prepared yourself adequately.

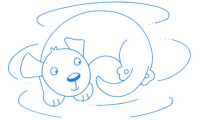

If you ticked most of the B boxes, you are probably quite absorbed in your studies and already have a well-developed deep and strategic approach to your learning. You should be in a good position to do well in your exams.

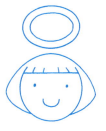

If you ticked most of the C boxes, you may not be very interested in what you are doing and perhaps time will slip by without you realising that you have not gained much from your studies. It would be a good idea to become more engaged and interested in the subject. You might start thinking about some questions to ask to help you.

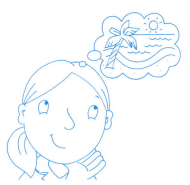

To summarise, so far we have looked at three aspects of learning:

1. extrinsic and intrinsic types of motivation

2. deep and surface approaches to learning

3. being strategic.

You have also had the opportunity to think about the kind of learner you are. This may feel as if you are being asked to fit yourself into a slot and forget about being an individual. But of course that is not the case!

There are two more aspects of learning to consider. Read on!

Being personally engaged and interested in learning, rather than being completely detached, makes it much easier to acquire new knowledge and to develop understanding. So studying effectively involves a combination of cognitive and affective aspects of our make-up (Bloom 1956a, 1956b).

Cognitive aspects of learning

On the cognitive side, it takes time to absorb and understand new and unfamiliar knowledge. But once it is fully grasped, it becomes possible to apply it, which is important for the OSCE. Trying to apply knowledge that has not been properly understood could have very negative consequences!

So, over to you!

ACTIVITY 3.6

Thinking about the cognitive aspects of learning, how are you studying for the OSCE? Jot down some points below.

....

....

....

....

....

....

For example, do you:

● Use a notebook to record the information that you feel is necessary for passing the OSCE – information like signs and symptoms of Type 1 diabetes, or a step-by-step procedure for hand-washing so that you can go over them repeatedly until you feel confident that you know it all?

● Study hypothetical situations of patients with certain symptoms, such as skin problems, and try to develop a list of possible nursing interventions related to these conditions?

● Study patient scenarios, such as family support and medical history, as a way of understanding health problems so that, when given a list of symptoms, you can ask questions to enhance your understanding of the patient's medical condition?

● Develop a checklist for the items that need to be covered to use for asking the necessary questions and interacting with a patient?

The kinds of learning strategies described above could be very helpful for moving you on.

The cognitive aspects of learning involve making sense of new knowledge to the extent that it can be used to gain more knowledge. What does this really mean? Perhaps you remember Figure 1.1 in Chapter 1. It shows how knowledge needs to be acquired and under-stood before it can be applied. To be successful in the OSCE, for every skill being examined, you need to apply your knowledge in the right way. This was represented by the arrows pointing upwards from the bottom to the top of the triangle.

In Figure 3.1 you will see that the arrows go downwards. This represents how development of the *cognitive* aspects of learning lead towards a bigger picture and shows how the mind of a deep and strategic learner develops. So here, in this figure, you can see that acquiring new knowledge is just the beginning of the learning journey.

Look at Step 1 at the top of the triangle. This part represents the new knowledge being learned. You will see that the next part, Step 2, is wider. This is all about understanding what the new knowledge really means. By thinking about new knowledge, it becomes more familiar, more significant and better understood. At Step 3, where the triangle is wider still, the understanding is good enough for the knowledge to

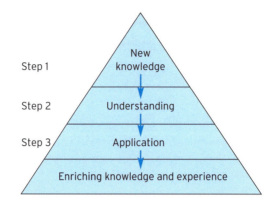

Figure 3.1 Developing the cognitive aspects of learning

be applied appropriately. By applying that knowledge, we extend our learning and gain more knowledge at a deeper level.

The point here is that, although application – the 'doing' of a skill – needs to be achieved, cognitive development should not stop there. Through our experiences, our thinking and our exposure to new situations, our knowledge is enriched and becomes deeper and broader. In fact developing new knowledge and understanding never ends! This is indicated in the bottom part of the triangle in 'enriching knowledge and experience'. What this really means is that, as we learn, we develop as critical thinkers who are able to analyse at least three things: the situations we find ourselves in, our actions, and the actions of others. We then have the capacity to develop our critical understanding of the world at a more abstract level and become able to make evaluative judgements about the ways things are done.

Let's pause for a moment to further consider the figure. One way of doing this is to relate its contents to a clinical skill. Familiarise yourself with the OSCE marking criteria for medication administration. (It is important to remember that this is just an example and that OSCE checklists will vary between colleges and universities.)

OSCE MARKING CRITERIA		
Oral medication		
Step	Yes	No
1 Check patient identification and allergies with prescription and name band	❏	❏
2 Identify medication prescribed	❏	❏
3 Identify date and time to be given	❏	❏
4 Check valid period	❏	❏
5 Check medication dose	❏	❏
6 Check route of administration	❏	❏
7 Check doctor's signature	❏	❏
8 Check expiry date on container	❏	❏
9 Dispense correct dose without contamination	❏	❏
10 Observe patient taking all prescribed medication	❏	❏
11 Check all pages of drug chart	❏	❏
12 Sign prescription accurately after giving medication	❏	❏

It could be argued that, if you are new to learning the skill of drug administration, all you need to know is the order of the procedure as identified in the 12 steps shown on the OSCE mark sheet. This would be the new knowledge, represented at the pinnacle of the triangle. What would be the limitation of this?

The answer would be that you undertook certain steps without knowing why. In other words you would be rote learning. You would have acquired new knowledge but cannot explain what it really means or indeed how to apply it.

Widening the triangle further to application, as an experienced nurse you will know that nursing is not linear. You would follow all the steps, but not necessarily in that order, and still maintain a safe procedure. For instance, you may not check the patient's identification band first because you know the patient. The order of your actions may be to prepare the medication, checking these details against the medication chart for the correctness of prescribing, and then check the name band at the point of administering the medicine.

Finally, if or because you have internalised the knowledge, you may start to question standard practice and generate new ideas to improve the process, such as implementing self-medication.

Affective aspects of learning

As human beings, our behaviour can be unpredictable because it partly depends on how we feel at the time. But thinking about the affective side of learning, with the OSCE in mind, may help to avoid unnecessary pitfalls.

ACTIVITY 3.7

So what are your strengths on the affective side? For example:

(a) When do you study best – in the morning, afternoon or evening?

(b) Do you feel confident and positive about working towards the OSCE?

(c) Are you a systematic worker?

(d) Have you started identifying the aspects of the OSCE that you are likely to perform well in, and those aspects where you need to improve?

(e) Do you feel a sense of commitment towards nursing or midwifery as a profession and being a health professional?

Think about these and jot down some answers/your notes below.

(a) ....

(b) ....

(c) ....

(d) ....

(e) ....

Being willing to learn is obviously the first requirement. Adopting a positive, receptive attitude towards learning new and unfamiliar concepts leads to an appreciation of their importance, not only in a particular context but also in a more general way. For example, the precise way in which a patient's temperature should be taken needs to be valued because of the possible range of consequences.

Figure 3.2 shows how the affective side is an essential part of learning. You will notice that the triangle is very similar to the triangle

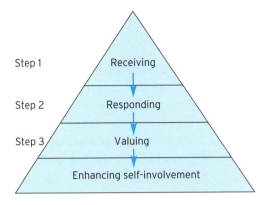

Figure 3.2 Developing the affective aspects of learning

in Figure 3.1 showing the cognitive side of learning. Figure 3.2 focuses on the *affective* side of learning. Here, Step 1 is about being willing to receive new information and this is represented at the top of the triangle. This willingness paves the way for Step 2, represented by a wider part of the triangle. Step 2 is about actively responding to what is being studied – being able to consider how to perform certain tasks such as wound care or to internalise factual information such as blood results or the causes of diabetes. Moving deeper, Step 3 is represented by the further widening of the triangle. At this point the information becomes more important: for example, why it is important or even necessary to dress a wound in the correct way? Being able to value the worth of that knowledge means that it becomes possible to apply it in the right way and under the best conditions, which is essential to demonstrate in an OSCE.

For many practitioners, receiving new information and/or changing how we practice nursing or midwifery is not easy, while for others it represents an opportunity to grow and develop. A willingness to learn is essential for receiving new information. How we apply this to learning for the OSCE can be well illustrated by the skill of communication. Nurses and midwives are skilled communicators but, with changes to practice or the context in which we work, we may need to broaden and develop our communication skills. If this is not achieved, a barrier to learning develops. This becomes relevant when thinking about OSCE success because a pre-registration nurse or midwife, and indeed a qualified nurse or midwife, may need to learn a new way of communicating even if they already think of themselves as good com-municators. Valuing new skills enables the application of those skills. This, in turn, enables valuing the application of those skills so that the practice itself is enabled to continually change and evolve.

But intrinsic motivation develops our affective side to an even higher and deeper level where we really make the most of our learning experiences, not only of our knowledge and understanding of the world around us but also of our self-knowledge and self-understanding: our own feelings and reactions in different situations. This is indicated in the bottom part of the triangle by 'enhancing self-involvement'. We become better able to appreciate the value of various skills, tasks and other elements within a certain situation. We develop our under-standing of the relationships among them so that we organise and prioritise them according to their value. In these ways we strengthen our sense of commitment and dedication to professional needs.

By now you may have realised that developing these cognitive and affective aspects of learning must automatically be empowering and confidence-building. They pave the way for lifelong learning.

Now – what about you?

ACTIVITY 3.8

These questions may help you to think about getting ready for the OSCE.

Do you feel:	Yes	No	Not sure
1. Positive about acquiring new knowledge?	❏	❏	❏
2. Able to fully value what you are learning?	❏	❏	❏
3. Confident about preparing for the OSCE?	❏	❏	❏
4. A sense of a sense of commitment about the OSCE?	❏	❏	❏
5. Enthusiastic about undertaking OSCE-type tasks?	❏	❏	❏
6. Able to handle unexpected situations?	❏	❏	❏

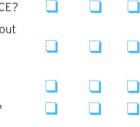

At present, you may not be able to answer 'yes' to all these questions. But at least they will help you to think about the affective side of the OSCE.

Preparing for the OSCE is not a night-before-the-event exercise! Thinking about all the aspects of learning covered in this chapter will help you to understand and enhance your own development, and the ways you prepare for the OSCE and beyond. Let's recap quickly what those aspects of learning are:

● intrinsic motivation

● deep learning

● strategic learning

● cognitive and affective aspects of learning.

In summary, learning comprises the interaction of cognitive and affective aspects of behaviour. These aspects can be developed through deep learning, being intrinsically motivated and adopting good strategies.

Let's think ahead to the OSCE itself, and get ready for Chapter 4, which is about preparing for the OSCE.

What is the examiner looking for?

You may remember thinking about the examiner's role in the OSCE earlier, in Chapter 1.

ACTIVITY 3.9

Do you need to know what the examiner is looking for? Think about this and write down a few notes below.

....

....

....

....

....

....

If your response to the question above is 'No', perhaps you should think again! Read on!

If your response to the question above is 'Yes', then the next question is 'Why?' Which is the best answer?

A. I can perform more confidently.

B. It helps me to understand the purpose of the OSCE.

C. It helps me to understand the examiner's role.

All three answers are good. Being confident during the OSCE is very important but it depends on being prepared in many aspects. Understanding the role of the examiner is important on an interpersonal level. In other words, it is a good guide for how you will need to behave and communicate during the OSCE. But this is only one part of understanding the purpose of the OSCE.

ACTIVITY 3.10

What exactly is the examiner's position in the OSCE? Think about this for a few minutes and write down some ideas below.

....

....

....

....

....

....

The examiner has a very important role in the OSCE. Her role is to assess how well you perform in the OSCE in light of the high standards of the profession.

Study hints and tips for the OSCE

- Begin preparing for the OSCE as soon as you can and think of it as a step-by-step process of your own development.

- Become engaged in your learning by exploring what is interesting about each topic and questioning things you don't understand.

- Get to understand yourself as a learner who is in the process of becoming a professional nurse.

- Find out how you learn best: on your own, and/or with others in a study group.

- Remember that the safest approach is a deep, strategic approach.

- Be a cue-seeker and capitalise on every opportunity to find out as much as you can about the OSCE.

- Become a deep thinker by exploring the underlying reasons for any situation you encounter.

- Practice the skills you need until they become second nature to you.

- Avoid getting too tired by spending long hours on your studies without a break.

- Try to visualise what will happen during the OSCE and rehearse it in your mind, not just once but several times.

Recap and recall

You have now reached the end of this chapter and you should have a sound understanding of what being an effective learner entails, why the OSCE is important, and how to approach it. To check your understanding of the key points we have covered, spend some time asking yourself the following questions:

- Do I know how to learn effectively so that I can prepare for the OSCE?

- Can I explain why preparing for the OSCE is important?

- Do I have an understanding of the key aspects of effective learning:
  - intrinsic motivation
  - deep learning
  - developing good learning strategies
  - combining cognitive and affective aspects of learning?

- Can I identify my strengths and needs in preparing for the OSCE?

Quick quiz

You might also like to test your knowledge and understanding with this quick quiz. You will find the answers at the end of the book.

Multiple choice

Choose the best answer from the options provided.

1. To have the best chance of passing the OSCE, which of the following preparation strategies is the most effective?

   A. Coping with the course requirements

   B. Being interested in the course content

   C. Asking as many questions as possible about the exam

   D. Memorising as many facts as possible

   E. Preparing for as many hours per day as possible

2. Which of the following is most like preparing for an OSCE?

   A. Working up an appetite

   B. Completing a jigsaw

   C. Predicting the future

   D. Trying to win a race

   E. Burying your head in the sand

3. Thinking about nursing and midwifery as a professional requires all the following apart from one. Which one?

   A. A strong empathy with people in general

   B. A desire to feel needed

   C. An ability to code-switch

   D. A strong sense of duty

   E. Having a good memory

True or false

Identify whether the following statements are true or false.

4. The cognitive and affective domains are equally important.

True ☐   False ☐

5. A strategic approach to learning is the passport to success.

True ☐   False ☐

6. A surface approach to learning will ensure a bare pass.

True ☐   False ☐

7. Perfecting skills is an essential part of preparing for the OSCE.

True ☐   False ☐

8. Preparing for the OSCE simply means taking a basic common-sense approach.

True ☐   False ☐

Matching pairs

Make six meaningful sentences by matching each item in the left-hand column with the most appropriate item in the right-hand column.

Being a good cue-seeker requires . . .	finding out how to pass the OSCE.
Taking a deep approach to learning means . . .	the best chances of success.
Being extrinsically motivated means . . .	thinking about some key questions to ask.
Being intrinsically motivated requires . . .	becoming stressed just before the OSCE.
Taking a surface approach to learning can lead to . . .	questioning new ideas and facts.
Taking a deep and strategic approach to preparing for the OSCE leads to . . .	being a deep learner.

Chapter 4

Preparation for the OSCE

'Success is a journey, not a destination.'

ARTHUR ROBERT ASHE, Tennis champion (1943-1993)

AIMS

At the end of this chapter, you should:

- Know what to expect from the OSCE
- Know how to prepare effectively for the OSCE performance
- Know how to maximise your chances of success

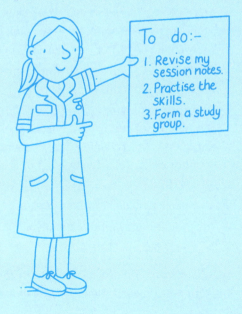

What you know at this stage

The first three chapters in this book will have given you some under-standing of OSCEs. Now spend a few minutes thinking about these questions:

- What is an OSCE?
- What actually happens during an OSCE?
- How is an OSCE assessed?

Jot down some ideas below.

Your answers should have included the following:

- An OSCE is a formal examination where you, the student, are expected to demonstrate certain clinical skills as well as the knowledge and attitudes underpinning those skills.
- OSCEs are as significant as other types of assessments such as written examinations and essays.
- Conventionally skills and knowledge are assessed during an OSCE at a number of stations. At each station, you are given a scenario with a task, which requires you to demonstrate a particular skill or set of skills. Collectively, a set of stations is referred to as a 'circuit'.
- An examiner/invigilator may or may not be present.
- The scenario may or may not involve a patient actor.
- Your performance is timed.

We will return to these points later in this chapter when considering the different types of scenarios you may encounter.

Essential elements of an OSCE

Knowing what an OSCE is and understanding the principles that underpin this method of assessment will help you to prepare for the exam.

In this section we will use three different OSCE scenarios to illustrate how the OSCE may apply at different levels of academic study, how OSCE stations may differ in terms of complexity, and how they are assessed. We will also discuss the type of preparation necessary to maximise your chances of success at each station.

The scenarios we will be looking at are:

- hand hygiene
- Body Mass Index (BMI) calculation
- assessment of the eye.

Before we look at each scenario, we need to consider three essential elements of all OSCE scenarios. These are *timing*, the *skills and knowledge* you are required to demonstrate during the OSCE, and your professional *attitude and behaviour*.

Timing

An essential feature of OSCEs is that they are timed. This means that, at each station, you will be given a set amount of time in which to demonstrate the required skill or skills. Depending on the nature of the task, the length of time may range from five minutes for a relatively simple skill, such as hand-washing, to up to an hour for a more complex scenario, which may comprise a set of skills with several integrated components. Importantly, as part of your preparation for the OSCE you will need to find out how many stations are included in the exam and the time allocated for your performance at each station.

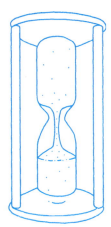

Demonstrating skill and knowledge

From reading Chapters 1 to 3, you will know that the main method of assessment used during an OSCE is observation. If an examiner is present at the station, he will always be watching you closely as you demonstrate the required skill. Additionally, you may be required to complete some form of documentation, such as an observation chart or wound care assessment tool, which will also be assessed.

It is important to understand, however, that a clinical skill requires more than just technical proficiency and consists of more than just the 'doing' part of the skill. In order to demonstrate competency, it is essential that you are also able to demonstrate the knowledge underpinning the skill. This part is often referred to as the cognitive or 'psycho' component. In fact, in the literature it is not uncommon to see clinical skills referred to as 'psychomotor skills' (Oermann 1990).

Your professional attitude and behaviour

This relates to the affective component. It is the way you act towards the person for whom and, if relevant, on whom you are performing the skill, i.e., the patient or client. The affective component also encompasses any safety or ethical issues associated with skill performance. If, for example, you were required to measure an adult's temperature using a tympanic ther- 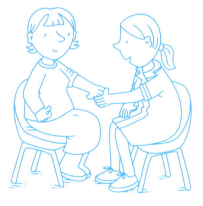 mometer, the examiner would be assessing not only your technical proficiency and skill with using the equipment and your knowledge of normal temperature ranges in adults, but also the way in which you interacted and communicated with the person while taking the temperature.

Knowledge, Motor skills, Attitude, Structure (KMAS)

Now that we have considered the essential elements of timing, skills, professional attitude and behaviour, we need to think about how they would apply to the OSCE in terms of the examiner assessing your performance. A useful way is to think of the main aspects of your performance that you must demonstrate. You may remember that these were introduced in Chapter 1. They include the knowledge (K) and understanding underpinning the skill; the motor skill (M) or technical aspects; the affective aspects, i.e., the professional attitude (A) associated with the performance; and finally (S) the structure, i.e., how the skill is demonstrated in terms of it being performed in a way that is both systematic and timely. The simple acronym KMAS may help you to remember these different aspects. Let's now look at three different scenarios in detail.

Example 4.1 Hand hygiene

This scenario involves hand washing, which is a relatively straightforward clinical skill that may be examined as part of an OSCE for first year pre-qualification nursing or midwifery students.

SCENARIO

You are preparing to give a patient an injection. Before starting you need to wash your hands.

Instructions: Demonstrate the recommended hand-washing technique.

Time available: 5 minutes.

ACTIVITY 4.1

Spend a few minutes considering what you are being asked to do at this station. Think about the technical and structural aspects as well as the knowledge and attitude required for effective demonstration of the skill. What is the assessor looking for? You may find it useful to write some notes below. The KMAS acronym may be a helpful prompt.

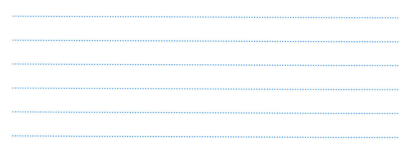

Compare your notes with the points below.

At this station you are being asked to decontaminate your hands within a five-minute time limit. To have adequately prepared for this station you would have revised your:

- **K (Knowledge and understanding of infection control)**: You should have revised the key principles of infection control and you will need to acknowledge that the hands of healthcare workers are implicated both in transmitting micro-organisms between patients and in spreading hospital-acquired infections. You should also know the appropriate times when it is necessary to wash or decontaminate your hands, and be able to list examples of such times. An understanding of the importance of each of the three stages involved in the hand-washing procedure is also necessary. These include preparation, washing and rinsing, and drying.

- **M (Motor skills)**: You should have practised your hand decontamination techniques and be able to demonstrate the recommended six-step hand-washing procedure. The examiner will be observing both your hand-washing technique and your ability to use the equipment without re-contaminating your clean hands when retrieving or discarding a used hand towel.

- **A (Attitude)**: You may think that a professional attitude has no relevance to hand hygiene, but this is not the case. Although hand-washing is not a skill that you will actually be performing on a patient, there are many situations when you will be washing or decontaminating your hands when you are in close proximity to patients or other members of the healthcare team. It is therefore essential that you are able to display a positive attitude towards this vital aspect of infection control.

- **S (Structure):** You should be able to perform the skill within the five-minute timeframe and demonstrate to the examiner a systematic and logical approach to the hand-washing process.

Example 4.2 Calculating a Body Mass Index (BMI)

This scenario is slightly more complex than the one illustrated in Example 4.1. You will see that the clinical skill that the student is required to demonstrate has more than one component.

SCENARIO

Mr Smith has been admitted for surgery. As part of his assessment, a Body Mass Index (BMI) needs to be measured.

Instructions: Mr Smith has been scheduled for surgery in the morning. As part of the pre-operative assessment process, you have been asked to calculate Mr Smith's BMI and to document the findings.

Time available: 8 minutes.

ACTIVITY 4.2

Consider what you are being asked to do at this station. Think about the four aspects, KMAS, which are all required for effective demonstration of the skill. What is the assessor looking for? Again, you may find it helpful to write some notes below.

Compare your notes with the points below.

To calculate a BMI you would need to measure the height and weight of Mr Smith. You would also need to perform a mathematical calculation and then document the result accurately. All this would have to be achieved within the eight-minute time limit.

To effectively prepare for this station you would have revised your:

- **K (Knowledge and understanding of BMI):** This includes knowing what a BMI is and the normal ranges of BMI. You should also be familiar with the metric system in order to obtain the correct type of data needed to perform the BMI calculation.

- **M (Motor skills):** You should have practised the technical skills required to accurately measure a patient's weight and height. This involves the ability to correctly use the equipment, i.e., a weighing scale and stadiometer.

- **A (Attitude):** Demonstrating a professional attitude is essential throughout this task. It is required when meeting and greeting the patient, obtaining consent, explaining the procedure and findings, and drawing the procedure to a close. This final part involves thanking the patient for his cooperation and checking that his needs are met.

- **S (Structure):** As with all OSCE stations, you will need to perform the skill within the allocated time limit. In this case this is eight minutes. Additionally, to demonstrate a structured and systematic approach, you will need to perform each of the components required to weigh and measure the patient in a logical order, so as to obtain the necessary data required to calculate the BMI while minimising any discomfort or inconvenience to the patient.

The examiner will observe you measuring and weighing Mr Smith to see that this is done accurately. The method you use to calculate the BMI will also be assessed to determine whether or not you are using the correct mathematical formula. The examiner will mark your documentation and your answer will be checked. Additionally, the way in which you interact and communicate with Mr Smith will be taken into consideration.

Example 4.3 Assessment of the eye

This example is more complex than Examples 4.1 and 4.2. It is likely to be a part of OSCEs for post-qualification nurses.

ACTIVITY 4.3

Consider what you are being asked to do at this station. Again, think about the four aspects, KMAS, which are all required for effective demonstration of the skill. You may find it helpful to write some notes below.

....

....

....

....

....

....

Compare your notes with the points below.

At this station you are being asked to take details from the patient and to examine a photograph of an eye showing signs of the symptoms the patient is describing. After ten minutes, a specific instruction is given by the examiner asking you to provide a differential diagnosis and to identify how this condition may be managed. You have been asked to complete this set of skills within a 20-minute timeframe.

To have prepared for this station you would have revised your:

- **K (Knowledge and understanding of the anatomy and physiology of the eye):** You will also require knowledge and understanding of the pathology of common eye conditions and an awareness and understanding of appropriate nursing management interventions and treatments.

- **M (Motor skills):** Although the skills required to complete this station are not technically motor in nature, you should have revised the skills necessary to obtain a relevant history from a patient and to provide feedback in a logical and systematic manner.

- **A (Attitude):** As with Example 4.2, demonstration of a professional attitude is an essential component of this skill and must be shown when meeting and greeting the patient, obtaining consent, explaining the procedure and findings, and bringing the episode to an effective close.

- **S (Structure):** As with the previous example, you will have a time limit for performing at this station when you will be required to undertake the patient assessment in a logical and structured way, using a systematic approach.

Example 4.3 is quite different from Examples 4.1 and 4.2 in terms of what the examiner will be assessing. The examiner will observe your attitude to the patient by watching for verbal and non-verbal communication skills. As you can see, you will also be assessed in terms of timeliness, efficiency and your ability to take a patient history within a specified period of time, which in this scenario is 20 minutes. The main part of the assessment, however, will involve listening to your feedback regarding the differential diagnosis and your discussion of nursing management interventions.

What does the examiner expect from you at the OSCE?

By this stage, you should feel more confident about the OSCE in terms of what is expected of you. But, to be on the safe side, let's think more deeply about this.

During the OSCE, the examiner will be assessing how well you translate knowledge, skills and attitude into action. The primary method of examination is usually by observation as seen in Example 4.1, the assessment of hand hygiene. However, you will also have noticed that Example 4.2, calculating a BMI, showed that the examination involved using a combination of observation, assessment of mathematical calculations, and accuracy of documentation. Example 4.3, which focused on eye assessment, was more demanding, in that the student had to obtain a patient history, verbalise her findings, make a differential diagnosis and discuss relevant nursing management interventions with the examiner.

Usually, during an OSCE, your performance will be assessed according to a checklist of criteria, which the examiner will use to gauge whether you have achieved the specific components that comprise the skill or set of skills. These are broken down into a sequence of steps, which make up the marking checklist. Here is an example checklist for hand-washing.

Step		Yes	No
1	Wets both hands thoroughly before applying hand-washing agent	❏	❏
2	Applies 2–3 squirts of hand-washing agent	❏	❏
3	Washes hands systematically	❏	❏
4	Washes both palms	❏	❏
5	Washes back of hand – right	❏	❏
6	Washes back of hand – left	❏	❏
7	Washes in between fingers of both hands	❏	❏
8	Washes backs of fingers – right	❏	❏
9	Washes backs of fingers – left	❏	❏
10	Washes around thumb joints – right	❏	❏
11	Washes around thumb joints – left	❏	❏
12	Washes fingernails/fingertips – right	❏	❏
13	Washes fingernails/fingertips – left	❏	❏
14	Completes handwash in 15–30 seconds	❏	❏
15	Rinses both hands thoroughly under running water	❏	❏
16	Turns taps off without contaminating hands	❏	❏
17	Retrieves hand towel without contaminating clean hands	❏	❏
18	Dries hands thoroughly including palms and backs of hands, between fingers and nails	❏	❏
19	Disposes of towel without contaminating hands	❏	❏

How to achieve a pass grade

If you have never done an OSCE before, you may be wondering how the marks are actually awarded, how many of the specific components of a skill you need to achieve on the marking checklist in order to pass a station, and what types of things may result in a fail grade. These are very relevant questions but, because of the wide variety of skills that can be assessed by means of an OSCE and the many different ways in which OSCEs can be conducted, it is important for you to discuss with your lecturers how the grades are calculated at your particular university or college.

Some key questions that would be helpful to ask are:

- Do I have to pass all stations within the circuit to pass the OSCE?
- Are there any 'killer stations' in the OSCE? You may remember that a 'killer station' refers to a station that **must** be passed in order to pass the OSCE.
- Do I have to achieve everything on the marking checklist to pass a station?
- Do any of the criteria on the marking checklist carry any bonus marks?

Being armed with the answers to these questions prior to the OSCE will help you to feel more confident and will assist with your preparation for the exam.

Conventionally, to be awarded a pass grade you will need to satisfy the examiner that you have fulfilled four key areas. Remember the KMAS acronym:

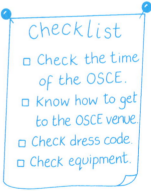

Checklist

☐ Check the time of the OSCE.
☐ Know how to get to the OSCE venue.
☐ Check dress code.
☐ Check equipment.

Knowledge and understanding

You will need to demonstrate the knowledge of how to undertake the skill from a technical perspective and show an understanding of the rationale underpinning the skill.

Motor skill

You will need to show that you can perform the skill in a technically proficient way.

Attitude

You will need to demonstrate safe and sensitive practice. In addition, you will be required to demonstrate professionalism with regard to your appearance, punctuality, your communication skills and the way in which you conduct yourself during the examination. You will need to identify and act on cues from the patient/client on whom or for whom the skill is being done.

Structure

You will need to perform the skill in a logical and systematic manner, paying adequate attention to detail. You will also need to complete the task within the given time constraints.

Why KMAS is important

A lack of attention to any of the above could potentially result in a fail grade being awarded. However, if your performance fulfils some of these criteria but not all and although you may not have done enough to convince the examiner that you are competent in all four areas, you may have done enough to be awarded a borderline grade. To explain what is meant by a borderline grade in more detail, let's now return to the hand-washing example.

As can be seen on the marking sheet shown previously, one of the steps requires the demonstration of a systematic approach to hand-washing. As recommended in the six-step hand-washing procedure advocated by many hospitals and healthcare settings, this approach involves washing the palms initially, followed by the backs of the hands, then between the fingers, the backs of the fingers, then the thumbs and finally the nails. This method of hand-washing can help to minimise the risk of missing any part of the hands. This is very important because any part of the hands may be contaminated with harmful micro-organisms.

Not following this recommended method when washing the hands is not in itself incorrect. However, it may be that a systematic technique is not used and this could jeopardise the skill being performed properly. For example, a student may start the procedure by washing their thumbs, followed by their nails. It is easy to see how the student may become a little muddled, forget which parts of their hands they have washed and repeat some of the previously performed steps or miss others. Demonstrating such a technique would not mean automatic failure of the OSCE station but the performance would not fulfil the four points the examiner is looking for. Let's remind ourselves what these involve in light of the student's performance in this example.

- **K (Knowledge and understanding):** In this example a general knowledge and understanding of hand decontamination has been demonstrated by the student but the examiner would note the lack of detail as the recommended six-step technique has not been followed.

- **M (Motor skill):** All parts of the hand need to be washed thoroughly to ensure that all surfaces of the hand are included. The student needs to demonstrate that she is using an effective technique.

- **A (Attitude):** As we noted earlier, attitude may not need to be assessed at this station but a positive and conscientious approach to hand decontamination by the student could be noted.

  The requirements for professionalism could be noted in the demonstration of safe and sensitive practice. Wearing the correct attire and removing any wristwatches or jewellery that may impede the hand-washing process would meet the requirements for professionalism.

- **S (Structure):** Demonstrating a muddled approach equates to parts of the performance being disorganised, even though the student could still demonstrate accuracy if all parts of the hands were effectively washed.

As can be seen, such a performance is likely to be assessed as 'borderline'. The student would have achieved some of the essential elements in terms of engagement and professionalism but the demonstrated performance would be weak with regard to the criteria of understanding and structure.

ACTIVITY 4.4

Consider the performances of two candidates, A and B, at the OSCE station presented below.

SCENARIO

John was discharged from hospital a month ago and is now under the care of his local community mental health team. He is managing well at home, his psychosis is controlled by medication and he is currently symptom-free. John has presented at the team base asking to see someone as his case worker is away. He is extremely concerned about a steady weight gain and wants to talk to someone about this. You have been asked to see him.

Instructions:

- Facilitate an interaction with John to explore his concerns.
- Formulate a short-term plan of action with John to address his concerns.
- Explain your rationale for the action plan to the examiner.

Time available: 20 minutes.

Candidate A

Candidate A greets John, sits down and immediately starts the interaction by exploring why John has come to the clinic. During the interaction Candidate A feels too far away from John and moves closer. John feels alarmed and moves his chair back. The candidate continues to give advice despite John saying that he doesn't understand. Throughout the interaction Candidate A does not make eye contact with John or display any warmth or understanding.

Candidate B

Candidate B introduces herself to John and checks that John is comfortable in terms of the environment where they are both sitting and their proximity to one another. The candidate explains to John that she is the duty nurse who will talk with him, before clarifying how *long they have for the interview. She then asks John to explain why he has come. After listening to John, Candidate B summarises his concerns before identifying a list of priorities to be addressed. These are shared with John and form the basis of the interview. The interview is closed.*

Look at the examiner mark sheet provided below, and consider both performances. Do you think Candidate A or Candidate B is most likely to be awarded a borderline grade?

OSCE MARKING CRITERIA		
Communicating with a patient		
Step	Yes	No
1 Sets up interview appropriately: checks environment is comfortable and private	❏	❏
2 Sets up interview appropriately: introduces self and role clearly	❏	❏
3 Sets up interview appropriately: states purpose of interview and gives timescale	❏	❏
4 Sets up interview appropriately: checks patient consent and understanding	❏	❏
5 Speech is clear and comprehensible: avoids frequent hesitation or rephrasing	❏	❏
6 Speech is clear and comprehensible: avoids jargon	❏	❏
7 Speech is clear and comprehensible: avoids multiple questions	❏	❏
8 Non-verbal behaviour conveys warmth and interest: open body posture	❏	❏
9 Non-verbal behaviour conveys warmth and interest: appropriate eye contact	❏	❏
10 Uses open and closed questions appropriately: uses a mixture of questions	❏	❏
11 Conveys understanding by: rephrasing questions	❏	❏
12 Conveys understanding by: summarising what the patient has said	❏	❏
13 Shows warmth and sensitivity by: reflecting back feelings as well as facts	❏	❏
14 Shows warmth and sensitivity: acknowledges client's viewpoint as important	❏	❏
15 Appears organised: covers agenda as set out at start of interview	❏	❏
16 Appears organised: is able to return to agenda appropriately if interaction digresses	❏	❏
17 Closes interview appropriately: indicates when interview is about to end	❏	❏

Step		Yes	No
18	Closes interview appropriately: seeks comments and questions from patient	❏	❏
19	Closes interview appropriately: thanks patient	❏	❏
20	Closes interview appropriately: summarises key issues from interview	❏	❏
21	Closes interview appropriately: indicates a future plan of action	❏	❏
22	Explains rationale for action plan to the examiner	❏	❏

ACTIVITY 4.5

Complete the table below by identifying key elements of both candidates' performance.

Candidate A	Candidate B
Knowledge and understanding:	Knowledge and understanding:
Achieved / Not achieved	Achieved / Not achieved
Motor skills:	Motor skills:
Achieved / Not achieved	Achieved / Not achieved
Attitude and professionalism:	Attitude and professionalism:
Achieved / Not achieved	Achieved / Not achieved
Structure:	Structure:
Achieved / Not achieved	Achieved / Not achieved

Did you rate Candidate A's performance as borderline? Although some of the key elements of the skill were demonstrated, you can see that a lack of attention to structure, empathy and professionalism marred his performance.

How do you feel about doing an OSCE?

So far in this chapter we have discussed in detail what is expected from you as a student during an OSCE. We have also looked at how OSCEs are assessed and we have briefly identified ways in which the marks and grades can be awarded. Let's now consider how you are feeling about OSCEs and what your expectations of the experience may be.

It is well known that OSCEs are a source of anxiety for many students, and you may be feeling quite nervous just reading this book and thinking about the OSCE and the sorts of things that you might be asked to do. However, everyone is different and you may, conversely, be feeling quite calm or even a little excited about the opportunity to demonstrate your clinical skills in a formal examination setting.

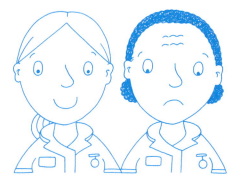

ACTIVITY 4.6

In order to discover more about your perceptions of OSCEs, select the statement below that best describes how you usually react in examination situations.

A. My nerves get out of control before exams and I am worried that this has a negative effect on my performance. ❏

B. A few pre-exam nerves are good for me as they help to keep me focused. ❏

C. I rarely get nervous before exams as I always make sure that I have studied hard and am very well prepared. ❏

D. I never feel nervous before exams as they really don't matter that much to me. ❏

As this activity is based on your own thoughts and feelings, there is no right or wrong answer but it is interesting to look at the response that you chose. Was it A or B? As we have previously discussed, many students do feel a little worried about OSCEs and this is quite natural. However, it is important that you have a plan in place that will help to keep your nerves in check so that you avoid panicking and stay calm during the exam. This may involve very simple strategies such as taking a few deep breaths before you begin each station or spending a few minutes alone mentally preparing yourself before entering the venue where the OSCE is to be held. If you are feeling particularly nervous, in the lead-up to the OSCE you may find it useful to engage in some relaxation exercises or spend time visualising the OSCE and thinking about what you may be asked to do. This could be a helpful way of alleviating some of your apprehension.

If you chose response C or D, it would seem that pre-examination nerves are not really an issue of concern for you. Although this may be good in some respects as it is unlikely that your nerves will get the better of you during the exam, it is important to avoid becoming over-confident because this could lead to inadequate time spent revising. OSCEs should be treated as seriously as all the other types of examinations and assessments that you will be required to do throughout your studies. So, having a structured revision plan that you stick to in the lead-up to the OSCE will enhance your chances of success.

Preparation is key to success!

Throughout this chapter we have emphasised the need to prepare thoroughly for your OSCE, just as you would for any other type of examination. As you will now recognise, OSCEs are often multi-dimensional and require demonstration of knowledge, motor skills and a professional attitude. As such, preparing for OSCEs will require a multifaceted approach. This may involve practising skills under supervision in the skills laboratory or with your mentor in the practice setting, revising your notes from relevant teaching sessions, under-taking recommended readings in journals, textbooks and websites, and engaging in mock OSCEs, or structured revision sessions. In summary, it is important to be prepared in order to:

● minimise stress and avoid panic
● understand fully what is required
● do everything that is required
● behave appropriately and professionally

- perform in an accurate, systematic and timely manner
- do full justice to your ability.

How to prepare for the day of the OSCE

It is useful to spend some time thinking about the best ways in which you can be prepared for the OSCE in order to maximise your chances of success. Perhaps you can reflect on other types of assessments and exams that you have recently done. How did you prepare for those? What worked best? How could your preparation have been improved?

Below are some suggestions for how to ensure that you are fully prepared on the day of the OSCE. You may also think of others, based on your own experiences.

- Predict what the OSCE will be like well in advance of the day.
- Become familiar with the OSCE process. This involves:
  - knowing what skills and knowledge may be examined
  - knowing how many stations there will be
  - knowing the duration of each station.

- Allow time to prepare mentally and physically on the day of the OSCE.
- Ensure you get a good night's sleep before the OSCE.
- Ensure you know where the OSCE will be held, and arrive on time.

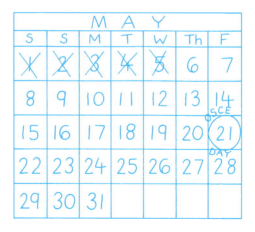

So let's think about this systematically. Advance thinking and planning can make all the difference to your OSCE day.

Countdown to the OSCE day

This is all about good time management!
What should you be doing and when?

From the beginning up to one month in advance

This is confidence-building time. So develop your clinical skills and acquire the knowledge and understanding you need to do well in the OSCE.

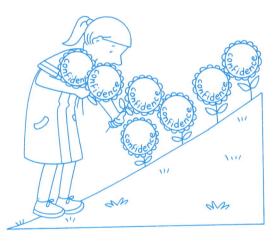

One month in advance

This is stock-taking time. Think about what you know and what you need to know. Do some enthusiastic cue-seeking. Ask yourself what further practice you need, what questions you now need to ask and how confident you now feel. Take advantage of any opportunity to get that practice. Plan your time carefully.

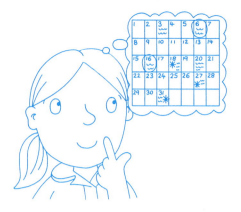

One week in advance

Now it is time to think about the OSCE experience: what it will be like and whether you feel ready for it. Address any last-minute doubts you might have by asking questions and checking your knowledge. Above all, remind yourself why the OSCE is so important. Try to visualise how you can do your very best in your appearance, behaviour, responses to what you are instructed to do and general professionalism. Practise frequently through mentally visualising and rehearsing the exam situation.

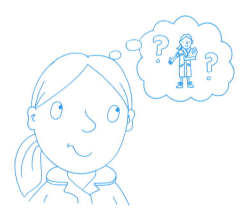

One day before

Be cool, calm and collected so that you can focus on the practical details. Check the time of the start of the exam, the exact venue, what you are going to wear and the time you need to be at the venue. Aim to arrive early so that you will feel as comfortable as possible to start the exam. Plan the journey to allow the maximum amount of time you need to get to the venue. You need to feel confident that you really will make it in good time.

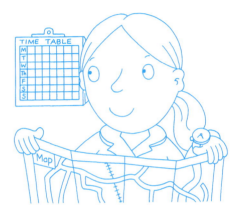

On the day!

Remember to allow time to prepare mentally and physically on the day.

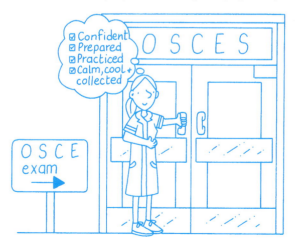

Recap and recall

You have now reached the end of this chapter. To check your understanding of the key points that we have covered, spend some time asking yourself the following questions:

- Do I know what an OSCE is?
- Do I understand what the examiner will be looking for and how my performance during the OSCE will be assessed?
- What are the best ways for me to prepare for the OSCE?
- Am I likely to have any specific problems? If so, what are these?
- What are my strengths and weaknesses?
- What strategies am I going to use to prevent my nerves getting the better of me during the OSCE?
- If I am not successful, what can I do to improve my performance?

Quick quiz

You might also like to test your knowledge and understanding with this quick quiz. You will find the correct answers at the end of the book.

Multiple choice

Choose the best answer from the options provided.

1. What do the letters in the acronym KMAS stand for?

A. Knowledge, Motor Skill, Attitude, Structure
B. Knowledge, Motor Skill, Assertiveness, Structure
C. Knowledge, Mastery, Attitude, Sympathy
D. Knowledge, Mastery, Assertiveness, Sympathy

2. During an OSCE the examiner will be assessing how well you translate knowledge, skills and attitudes into an action that is:

A. Structured, timely and non-systematic
B. Structured, systematic but not timely
C. Timely, structured and systematic
D. Timely and systematic but not structured

3. On the day of the OSCE it is recommended that you are prepared:

A. Physically and financially
B. Mentally and physically
C. Mentally and financially
D. Mentally and logistically

4. The letter 'A' in the KMAS acronym refers to which of the following:

A. Action
B. Attention
C. Attitude
D. Assessment

True or false

Identify whether the following statements are true or false.

5. A useful strategy to ensure that you are fully prepared on the day of the OSCE involves predicting what the OSCE will be like well in advance.

True ☐   False ☐

6. OSCE examiners like to see students fail and will try to trick them during the exam.

True ☐   False ☐

7. It is well known that OSCEs are a source of stress and anxiety for many students.

True ☐   False ☐

8. Many students pass OSCEs by just studying the night before the exam.

True ❑   False ❑

9. Preparation is key to success in an OSCE.

True ❑   False ❑

Chapter 5

The OSCE experience

'Everyone who got where he is has had to begin where he was'.

ROBERT LOUIS STEVENSON, Novelist (1850–1894)

AIMS

At the end of this chapter you should:

- Have gained an insight into the OSCE experience from the perspective of students and examiners
- Be able to identify some top tips for success with your OSCE
- Be able to formulate a plan to assist you with your own OSCE preparation

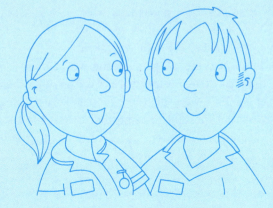

If you have read the previous chapters in this book you should now have a good understanding of what an OSCE is, typical ways in which an OSCE may be conducted and the types of skills and knowledge that may be assessed during this unique type of examination. However, you may also be interested in what the actual experience of doing an OSCE is like and, more importantly, what you can do to maximise your chances of success.

To consider these aspects and more, this final chapter will draw on the experiences of students and examiners who have been involved in the OSCE process. So, to learn more about the OSCE experience, read on.

What is it like to take an OSCE?

OSCEs are now used extensively in health education for all branches of nursing, midwifery and medicine, and for some students just the thought of having to do an OSCE may be daunting. To find out more, you may have already spoken with other students or practice colleagues about their OSCE experiences. They may have shared with you both positive and not-so-positive experiences. This is because, just like other types of assessment, OSCEs will appeal to 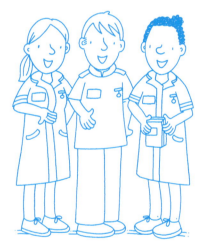 different types of learners and may be suited more to some people than to others. Furthermore, it is likely that those who have done well in an OSCE will view them more favourably than those who haven't. What is important to remember is that the OSCE is a very individual experience. However, there are things that you can do to help maximise your chances of success.

The student perspective

Let's take a look at what some students had to say about their experience with OSCEs. You will see that these students are all different in terms of their programmes, experiences and the level at which they are studying. However, there are also some important themes.

'An OSCE can be a bit nerve-racking, just like any other exam, however, the main thing is not to panic and to focus on what you are doing, and of course, to read the instructions carefully. You will find some stations harder than others, just like exam questions, and the main thing is to complete each station and then move on. When the results came out, some people were surprised at how well they did, so it is important to give each station your all, regardless of how you feel the previous one went.' (3rd year adult branch nursing student)

'The exam is very formal, and I didn't expect that. You are not allowed to talk to any of the other students although you may be hanging around outside the stations together for a few minutes. I wanted to tell the other students what to expect, and also to hear from them what the next station was, but the formal nature of the exam means strictly no talking.' (2nd year mental health branch nursing student)

Now over to you!

ACTIVITY 5.1

Having read some accounts by students of their OSCE experiences, how do you feel about OSCEs now? What hints can you pick up from these comments that may help you? Jot down some notes below.

Both students indicate the formal nature of an OSCE (which was descri-bed in Chapter 4). The second student, however, makes an important point. She was tempted to tell other students the content of the OSCE. But remember that an OSCE is an exam and this could constitute cheating. On a personal level, you have worked for the exam and your performance is the result of your own efforts. On a practical level, stations are often changed between examining students to prevent disclosure.

Here are comments from two more students.

'During the exam, if things go badly at one station, just keep going and try to do as well as you can at the next one. It is hard not to think about the mistakes that you may have made previously, but try to put these out of your head, and focus on the task in hand.'

(Qualified nurse studying at post-graduate level)

'I felt most nervous when I was outside waiting to go into the OSCE. I kept going through in my head all the things I had learnt, and tried to stay calm. When the exam started, I was still very nervous, but it wasn't nearly as bad as I had imagined. I made a point of explaining out loud what I was doing, and talked to the actor, as though they were a real patient in the ward. I soon almost forgot that it was an exam and I was being assessed.' (Midwifery student)

You may have noticed that all these students mention possible pitfalls but make some constructive comments about moving forward. So their general message is to stay focused and positive!

Your OSCE preparation

Throughout this book, we have emphasised the importance of prepar-ing well for the OSCE and, if you have read the previous chapters, you will be well on the way to knowing what OSCE preparation entails. Indeed, it may be that you have already started your own preparation. It is also very likely that any students or lecturers to whom you may have spoken about OSCEs will also have talked about the importance of good preparation. But remember, there is no one correct strategy regarding OSCE preparation that will guarantee success. How you prepare will depend on a number of different factors. In fact, you may use a variety of approaches. These may be dependent on the following:

- the type of learner you are
- the length of time you have to prepare for the OSCE
- the type of OSCE you will have
- the types of skills and knowledge that you may be assessed on
- the type of study support you may have including friends, colleagues and clinical mentors
- the types of resources available to you.

At the end of the book you will find a personalised OSCE preparation plan for you to fill in as you get ready for your exam.

Here students share with you some of their OSCE preparation strategies.

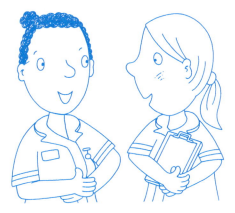

'I prepared by reading through the theory and making sure that my knowledge and understanding were up to date. I also practised with my friends on the course. I found sharing ideas and explaining how to do something to others really increased my confidence and ability.'

(Adult branch nursing student)

'I actually drew pictures of each skill that I thought I might be examined on. I then labelled them so that I had a visual reference – when learning a skill, I think you need to use visual prompts. For example, you see hand gel and remember to wash you hands.'   (Adult branch nursing student)

'Just reading books and articles didn't work for me. I found it most helpful to imagine myself performing each step of the skill, whenever

I had a chance. This could be on the bus, on a walk – wherever! Doing this really helped to cement the skill for me.'

(Adult branch nursing student)

'Initially, I wrote down all the steps of each potential OSCE skill. I then transferred these written steps to a visual image in my mind and started to visualise myself physically doing each step. It is these images that I returned to over and over again as I prepared for the OSCE. If I had a problem visualising a particular task, I then rectified this by actually performing the skill in either the clinical skills lab or the placement area.'

(Child branch nursing student)

'I used all the resources that were available to me – my notes, the online formative activities and the revision sessions. I also formed a study group with my peers. This was especially helpful because, as a group, we were able to exchange any notes we had made in the skills sessions, and practise together in the clinical skills room.'

(Post-qualification nursing student)

'As a mental health student, I found that there were limited oppor-tunities to practice clinical skills, especially during the Common Foundation Programme (CFP). This worried me a bit so, while on placement, I told my mentor that I had to sit an OSCE. He was really helpful and we spent a lot of time going through the skills. He even allowed me to practise blood pressure measurement on him and some of the other nurses.' (Mental health branch nursing student)

'With some friends, we booked some time in the skills centre, and set up a station, similar to that we expected would be in the exam. For example, we set up a urinalysis station, with all the essential equipment such as apron, gloves, alcohol hand gel, urine testing sticks, and the chart to write the results. We took turns timing each other and at the end, each member of the group received feedback from the others. I made a note of the comments they made and the things I needed to improve.'

(CFP nursing student)

Your turn now!

ACTIVITY 5.2

You will note that each of the OSCE preparation strategies described by students was quite different. None are right or wrong but each illustrates how different we all are as learners. In the space below, jot down some notes about things that you can do that you think will help you to prepare for the OSCE. You may wish to refer back to Chapters 1 and 3 to help you with this.

Ten top tips from students

Over the years we have worked with many students at all levels of study and the following themes keep recurring:

1. Rehearse, rehearse, rehearse!
2. Form a study group.
3. Find out what resources your university offers, for example, online tutorials, web packages and/or independent study facilities.
4. Access resources early on.
5. Think about your approach to study and what works best for you.
6. Enlist the help of family and friends.
7. If you are in practice, seek the help of your mentor.
8. Use your lecture notes.
9. Remember it is a formal exam.
10. Arrive on time and try not to panic.

You will now appreciate that there are many ways to prepare for an OSCE, and the method you choose will reflect the type of learner you are and how you learn best. Let's now turn our attention to the OSCE examiner.

The examiner's perspective

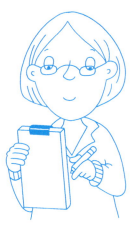

It is worth remembering that, contrary to what some students may think, OSCE examiners and lecturers have your best interests at heart. As such, they want you to be successful in the OSCE and are not out to trick you, nor do they want to see you fail. However, it is also important to remember that examiners have an important role to fulfil in relation to OSCEs and that is to accurately and fairly assess each student's level of proficiency and knowledge regarding a particular task or skill. Clearly, this is crucial for ensuring students are fit for practice and possess the skills and knowledge required to provide safe, good quality patient care.

By now you will recognise that OSCEs can be used as a formal type of assessment and are considered as important as written examinations, essays or presentations. As such, this requires focus and concentration on the part of the examiner. Therefore, do not expect the examiner at the OSCE station to engage in general conversation or any informal chit-chat with you before, during or after you have completed the required skill or task. Even if you know the examiner from your lectures or classes, it is likely that, during the OSCE, they will adopt a more formal and professional approach than you are used to.

Now let's read what some examiners have to say about OSCEs.

A very experienced lecturer made the following comments:

'I have been examining OSCES in nursing for many years and recognise that most students will be nervous. In fact, I would go so far as to say that I would find it unusual if a student undergoing an OSCE was not nervous. In this way an OSCE can be regarded as a level playing field. My advice for students would be to anticipate their nerves and to try to develop strategies to help cope with these before they begin. This could be as simple as taking a deep breath or silently repeating a positive mantra before starting. It has been my experience over and over again

that those students who are able to control their nerves and just get on with the task at hand are more likely to succeed than those who crumple up and let the nerves take over!' (Adult nurse lecturer)

Other comments made by the following lecturer highlight the differences between those students who are prepared for the OSCE and those who are not.

'I am an experienced lecturer who regularly examines student midwives undertaking OSCEs. From my perspective, it is really clear to distinguish between those students who have prepared for the OSCE, and those who haven't. Those who have prepared know what they are doing. They usually demonstrate a systematic approach to the task at hand, and although they may be nervous, it is evident that they have practised the skill and also studied the underlying theory. On the other hand, students who are unprepared are generally all over the place. They may start off okay, but then usually panic and start to make mistakes as they realise they are running out of time.' (Midwifery lecturer)

Again, the following comments demonstrate the importance of preparation and communicating with the examiner if things aren't going smoothly.

'If a student knows how to perform a skill, they will show it and it soon becomes very clear which students don't know what they are doing! My advice to students is that, if things are not going right during the OSCE station, let the examiner know. At least this way, they will know that you are safe.' (Mental health lecturer)

ACTIVITY 5.3

What key messages regarding the OSCE can you take from the examiners' comments above? Write some notes below.

....

....

....

....

....

....

Perhaps you have noticed from these comments that the examiners are very observant. If you haven't prepared sufficiently, they will notice. You cannot pull the wool over their eyes!

Ten top tips from examiners

As lecturers who have been involved in the development, organisation and examination of nursing and midwifery OSCEs for many years, we have witnessed at first hand students who perform poorly in OSCEs due to a lack of adequate preparation or because they do not conduct themselves as expected during the examination. Our ten top tips for success are:

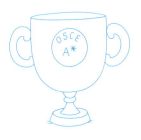

1. Remember that an OSCE is a formal examination. The examiner will be formal and will expect you to behave in a formal way too. Don't expect the examiner to engage in informal conversation with you.

2. Read the scenario and the relevant instructions carefully and think about what you are being asked to do. Don't be too impulsive or make assumptions about the task before reading both the scenario and the instructions thoroughly.

3. Ensure that your appearance is smart and tidy, and that it reflects professional standards. If you are required to wear a uniform, this should be clean and ironed. Appropriate footwear should be worn and attention paid to personal grooming and jewellery in line with regulations set by your college, university or Trust.

4. Keep to the time limit by timing your performance carefully. It is essential to wear a watch during the OSCE.

5. Use all the time allotted to demonstrate your performance skill to the best of your ability. If you finish demonstrating the required skill before the allocated time is up, use the remaining time wisely. Sit quietly and think about your performance. Have

you missed anything or is there anything you need to tell the examiner before moving on to the next station?

6. If the examiner uses set prompts or questions, respond to them.

7. Keep going even if you think you have performed poorly at a particular station or in an element of a complex scenario. Remember that your perception could be quite different from the examiner's observations.

8. If you realise you have just made a mistake, be open about it. Correct it and explain what you are doing and why.

9. If the scenario involves a patient actor with whom you are required to communicate, remember to bring the episode to an effective close by thanking the patient/client and checking that her needs have been met.

10. Try to avoid analysing your performance with your fellow students after the examination. Although tempting, this often leads to unnecessary stress and anxiety.

Avoiding common pitfalls

To maximise your success in the OSCE it is important that you avoid some common pitfalls that may negatively affect your preparation and performance on the day.

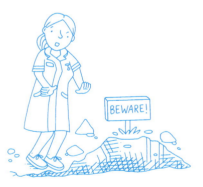

First, you are bound to feel nervous prior to the examination. So try not to add to those nerves by not being in control. Instead, take control! This is how.

● Plan your journey to the examination venue. You may be travelling to a new venue for the first time or to a familiar venue but at an unusual time.

● Leave plenty of time for your journey so that you arrive well before the start of the OSCE.

- Make sure you have the necessary requirements to enter the exam, i.e., your examination number.

- Ensure you have a pen that works and any other equipment you may need: e.g., a watch with a second hand.

- When entering each station never assume that what you are being asked to do is obvious. Read the scenario and instructions carefully each time.

- Make full use of your allotted time at every station.

- Adopt a professional approach when communicating with the examiner and patient role players. Remember that an OSCE is a formal assessment.

Second, you may recall the section on learning approaches in Chapter 3. If you are only a surface learner, remember that this will be a significant barrier to achieving success at your OSCE. At best you are likely to be a borderline student because you will have just rote-learnt a skill without understanding the principles underlying it. But worse, you are in danger of failing. Try not to be a surface learner who:

- has not attempted to understand the rationale for the OSCE as a whole and in its constituent parts,

- has not appreciated the need for thorough preparation in advance,

- is interested only in getting through the OSCE day,

- is unable to respond adequately to the instructions and the examiner's comments.

What does it feel like to be unsuccessful in an OSCE?

You might be interested in exploring what it feels like to have to re-sit an OSCE. Although we are not recommending that you anticipate this will happen, many students who are unsuccessful at passing OSCEs on their first attempt use this as a useful learning experience. Do you want to find out more? Then read on.

It goes without saying that everyone likes to be successful, and if we are not successful in the things we set out to achieve we are usually left feeling low and negative. In fact, one of the most common responses by students on hearing that they have not passed an exam is to give up.

You may or may not have had experiences with failure in other types of exams and assessments. If you have, you will appreciate that one of the best things to do is to take some time to let the news sink in and then to seek help. Let's now take a look at what some students who did not pass their OSCEs had to say about this.

'When I found out that I had failed the OSCE, I took the news very badly. I was really worried about it – in fact, it ruined my summer as I knew that I had a re-sit at the end of August. However, this was a great motivator for me to really learn and practise the skills. I talked to my mentor and we agreed that I needed to spend some time practising skills and improving my confidence. She was really helpful and helped me to identify opportunities where I could do this. When I did the re-sit, things went much better and I really knew what I was doing.'

(2nd year adult branch nursing student)

'I felt dreadful when I saw that I had failed the OSCE. In fact, when I found out, I wanted to give up nursing altogether. However, I felt a bit better a few days later after talking with my friends and knew that I needed to be proactive if I wanted to pass. So, I went to see the course leader, who told me which stations I hadn't passed. Overall, I hadn't done as badly as I initially thought, and it was really helpful to know what skills I really needed to work on.'

(CFP nursing student)

'The first OSCE I took I failed. This was on TPR, and I had to take a patient's pulse and respirations and record them on a chart. I tried to describe the patient's pulse to the examiner before I wrote it down but this came out all muddled. Then the bell rang and I was out of time. I wasn't surprised when the results came out and I saw that I had failed.'

(Child branch nursing student)

'When I re-sat the OSCE exam, I was determined to pass. I had really prepared hard for it and don't think I could possibly have done anything else. I was still very nervous but made a point of talking to the examiner to explain everything I was doing. I was so relieved when I found out that

I had passed. Overall, the experience really taught me how important it was to be prepared for OSCEs.' (Post-qualification midwife)

If you have been unsuccessful at your OSCE and are reading this part of the chapter, you may be able to identify with some of the thoughts and feelings of the students above. Once you are feeling ready, try to adopt a positive approach as some of these students did. Remember you are not on your own. Learn from the experience, seek feedback, and identify the support available to you. Think about whether there were gaps in your knowledge. Plan your revision strategy carefully. You may find it useful to write an action plan. These kinds of strategies will help to maximise your chances of success.

Moving on from the OSCE experience

The OSCE is not the end, but the beginning! Whatever happened during the OSCE and however successful or unsuccessful you were, there is no doubt that the experience is a deeply formative one. In other words you will have learnt a great deal and can move on.

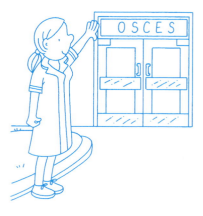

Think about this for a moment. You may already have faced some challenging situations in the past, so you may have an idea of how you will react after the OSCE.

Think about the following questions to help you move forward.

ACTIVITY 5.4

● How are you likely to react after your performance?

● How can your reactions be a constructive tool for moving on?

● What questions could you ask yourself after the event that would help you?

● In what sense is the OSCE the beginning and not the end?

You may find it useful to write some notes below.

....

....

....

....

....

....

You will appreciate that the OSCE can never be regarded as an isolated exam because it is fundamental to the whole context of your education. The skills that are being tested are crucial to your development as a health professional. So once you have recovered from the experience it is worthwhile putting it into a longer-term perspective. Your own actions and reactions during the OSCE may have surprised you in a positive or negative way. Whatever you feel, be constructive. Ask yourself how you can learn from it.

What happens if you are unsuccessful?

Of course, nobody wants to fail an OSCE. But if you happen to be unsuccessful you may need a little time to absorb what this means. It is most important to remember that this seemingly negative result is really in your own interest as well as in the interest of the whole profession. So you need to develop a positive frame of mind even if you feel like forgetting all about the experience. How can you do this? Well, there are two ways.

One way is to develop your self-knowledge and use that to your advantage. First, ask yourself what kind of person you were in the OSCE situation, how you personally reacted: whether you were confident, in control and able to concentrate on what you were doing or nervous and started to panic; whether or not you remembered everything you had learnt; whether you focused or became distracted by something. Remind yourself about the steps in the affective side of development shown in the triangle in Figure 3.2 in Chapter 3: being receptive to more knowledge, then being responsive to it, then valuing it and then enhancing your involvement. In this way you will develop a much stronger sense of what the OSCE entails as well as more confidence.

The second way is to develop your knowledge and understanding about the OSCE itself. Try to recall every station and every task that you were given. Ask yourself why you were given each one, what was being tested and why it was important.

ACTIVITY 5.5

How can you move on? Use the space below to jot down a few ideas.

....

....

....

....

....

....

By thinking of the OSCE as a formative experience, you are already moving closer to your goal of enhancing yourself professionally. There are several steps you can take to help yourself.

1. Ask yourself if you could have prepared more thoroughly in advance.

2. Deepen your understanding of the tasks you were required to perform at different stations by studying to increase your knowledge. For example, if, as part of an OSCE, you were required to assess a pressure ulcer and then choose an appropriate wound dressing based on your findings, it may be useful to expand your knowledge of wound care by reading about wound care management strategies.

3. Give yourself more practice to develop and refine your skills as far as you can so that they become second nature to you.

4. If you feel that you cannot identify what may have gone wrong, seek help at the earliest opportunity. Try to obtain as much detailed feedback on your performance as possible and make sure that you can understand it and identify with it. Writing an action

plan with the assistance of a personal tutor, lecturer or mentor may also be very useful.

5. Above all, remember that the skills that are examined in an OSCE are skills that you must acquire to a level that is clinically safe.

Some final comments: the OSCE rewards

Now that you have reached the end of this chapter, you will recognise that OSCEs are a unique type of clinical assessment that may be both challenging and rewarding, and of benefit to your practice. These sentiments are evident in the following student comments:

'The OSCE system is designed to challenge the student whilst providing the motivation to pass. While it was a huge challenge, when I look back, I can now see how beneficial doing the OSCE was to my overall confidence and preparation for practice.'

(First year adult branch nursing student)

'Doing an OSCE really did make a difference to my learning and practice. Passing the OSCE gave me a huge sense of pride in my practice.'

(3rd year child branch nursing student)

'I worked really hard for the OSCE and felt that I deserved to pass. It was worth all the effort.' (Post-qualification mental health nursing student)

'The course was essential for my career progression and therefore I had to pass the OSCE. It was such a relief to know that all my hard work had paid off and I had been successful.'

(Qualified midwife post-graduate study)

Recap and recall

You have now reached the end of this chapter and you should have a sound understanding of what being an effective learner entails, why the OSCE is important, and how to approach it. To check your understanding of the key points we have covered, spend some time asking yourself the following questions:

- Do I have greater insight into the OSCE experience from both a student and examiner stance?
- Can I list some of the top ten tips for success?
- Can I now identify some common pitfalls and do I know how to avoid these?
- Do I know how to move on from the OSCE experience?

Quick quiz

You might also like to test your knowledge and understanding with this quick quiz. You will find the correct answers at the end of the book.

Multiple choice

Choose the best answer from the options provided.

1. Preparation for an OSCE involves which of the following:

A. Recognising the type of learner you are

B. Understanding the type of OSCE you will take

C. Identifying the sources of support available to you

D. All of the above

2. During the OSCE the examiner is likely to:

A. Engage in informal, friendly conversation

B. Comment on your performance and how you are doing

C. Adopt a formal, professional approach

D. Provide you with answers and cues

3. If during the OSCE you realise that you have made a mistake, an effective strategy would be to:

A. Correct the mistake and explain what you are doing and why

B. Ignore the mistake and continue with the task

C. Try to hide the mistake by distracting the examiner

D. Give up and leave the OSCE

4. Which of the following is a common OSCE pitfall?

    A. Being well prepared and anticipating the skills you may be assessed on

    B. Ensuring you have all the necessary equipment with you

    C. Turning up on time to the OSCE venue

    D. Not utilising the time allocated to you at each station

True or false

Identify whether the following statements are true or false.

5. Preparing for the OSCE takes time and hard work, but the results are often very rewarding.

    True ❑   False ❑

6. Taking time to revise, practise and refine skills so that they become familiar is a useful preparation strategy for OSCEs.

    True ❑   False ❑

7. Analysing your performance with your fellow students after the examination often leads to unnecessary stress and anxiety.

    True ❑   False ❑

8. If you are unsuccessful in your OSCE it may be useful to write an action plan to help to identify and address key areas for development.

    True ❑   False ❑

Answers to Activities and Quick quizzes

Chapter 1

Answers to Activity 1.3
Example 1: Hand washing
Example 2: Post-partum assessment including accurate documentation of findings
Example 3: Nursing assessment and pain assessment

Answers to Quick quiz
1. B   2. D   3. A   4. B   5. True   6. False

Chapter 2

Answers to Activity 2.3
There are a number of errors and omissions on this chart. They are:

1. The respiratory rate for 1100hrs on the 10/9 is written in numerical format rather that being charted.
2. The respiratory rate is not documented for 1400hrs on the 10/9.
3. The blood pressure is written in numerical format (120/70) and charted for 2200hrs.
4. The pulse is recorded unclearly at 2200hrs.
5. The date is missing for the observations charted at 2200hrs.
6. Observations are not recorded for 1000hrs on the 11/9.

Answers to Quick quiz
1. A   2. B   3. B   4. D   5. True   6. True

Chapter 3

Answer to Activity 3.2

Learning behaviour	Surface	Deep
Intending to cope with the course requirements	☑	☐
Intending to understand ideas for oneself	☐	☑
Treating the course as unrelated bits of knowledge	☑	☐
Relating ideas to previous knowledge and experience	☐	☑
Looking for patterns and underlying principles	☐	☑
Memorising facts and procedures routinely	☑	☐

Answers to Quick quiz

1. B 2. C 3. B 4. True 5. False 6. False 7. True 8. False

Answers to Matching pairs

- Being a good cue-seeker requires thinking about some key questions to ask.
- Taking a deep approach to learning means questioning new ideas and facts.
- Being extrinsically motivated means finding out how to pass the OSCE.
- Being intrinsically motivated requires being a deep learner.
- Taking a surface approach to learning can lead to becoming stressed just before the OSCE.
- Taking a deep and strategic approach to preparing for the OSCE leads to the best chances of success.

Chapter 4

Answers to Quick quiz

1. A 2. C 3. B 4. C 5. True 6. False 7. True 8. False 9. True

Chapter 5

Answer to Quick quiz

1. D 2. C 3. A 4. D 5. True 6. True 7. True 8. True

My personal OSCE preparation plan

Use these pages to make notes to help you prepare for your OSCE. You may wish to photocopy them so you can reuse them.

Date and time of OSCE
Venue
My travel arrangements
Skills and knowledge likely to be assessed

Skills and knowledge I need to know

Study and preparation strategies

Resources available at my university that I can use to assist with my preparation

Other useful resources (websites, textbooks, journal articles)

My personalised preparation countdown plan

One month before the OSCE

-
-
-
-
-
-
-
-
-

One week before the OSCE

-
-
-
-
-
-
-
-

The day before the OSCE

-
-
-
-
-
-
-
-
-
-

The day of the OSCE

-
-
-
-
-
-
-
-
-
-

Contact details for study group members

Notes

References

Bloom, B.S. (1956a) *Taxonomy of Educational Objectives: Book 1 Cognitive Domain*. London: Longman.

Bloom, B.S. (1956b) *Taxonomy of Educational Objectives: Book 2 Affective Domain*. London: Longman.

Department of Health (2001) *Essence of Care. Patient Focused Benchmarks for Clinical Governance*. London: NHS Modernisation Agency.

Department of Health (2003) *Essence of Care. Patient Focused Benchmarks for Clinical Governance*. London: NHS Modernisation Agency.

Department of Health (2004) NHS Knowledge and Skills Framework (NHS KSF) http://www.dh.gov.uk/en/Publicationsandstatistics/Publications/PublicationsPolicyAndGuidance/DH_4090843.

Department of Health (2007) *Essence of Care. Patient Focused Benchmarks for Clinical Governance*. London: NHS Modernisation Agency.

Entwistle, N. (1997) 'Contrasting perspectives on learning', Chapter 1 in Marton *et al. The Experience of Learning: Implications for Teaching and Learning in Higher Education* (2nd edn). Edinburgh: Scottish Universities Press (pp. 3-22).

Entwistle, N.J. & McCune, V. (2004) 'The conceptual bases of study strategy inventories', *Educational Psychology Review* **16**, 325-346.

Infection Control Nurses Association (2003) *Infection Control Guidelines for General Practice*. London: ICNA.

Marton, F., Hounsell, D. & Entwistle, N. (1997) *The Experience of Learning: Implications for Teaching and Learning in Higher Education* (2nd edn). Edinburgh: Scottish Universities Press.

Miller, M.D. (1990) 'The assessment of clinical skills/competence/performance', *Academic Medicine* **65**(9), S63-S67.

NICE (2003) *Infection Control. Prevention of healthcare associated infection in primary and community care*. London: National Institute for Health and Clinical Excellence.

Nursing and Midwifery Council (NMC) (2004) *Midwives Rules and Standards*. London: NMC.

Nursing and Midwifery Council (NMC) (2007) *Essential Skills Clusters for Pre-registration Nursing Programmes*. NMC Circular 07/2007. http://www.nmc-uk.org/aDisplayDocument.aspx?documentID=3663.

Nursing and Midwifery Council (NMC) (2008a) *The Code: Standards of Conduct, Performance and Ethics for Nurses and Midwives*. London: NMC.

Nursing and Midwifery Council (NMC) (2008b) *Standards for Medicines Management*. London: NMC.

Nursing and Midwifery Council (NMC) (2009) *Guidance for Care of Older People*. London: NMC.

Oermann, M. (1990) 'Psychomotor skill development', *Journal of Continuing Education in Nursing* **21**, 202–204.

Rowntree, D. (1988) *Learn How to Study* (3rd edn). London: Macdonald & Co.

Royal College of Nursing (2005) *Good Practice in Infection Prevention and Control: Guidance for Nursing Staff*. London: RCN.

Rushforth, H. (2007) 'Objective structured clinical examination (OSCE): Review of literature and implications for nursing education', *Nurse Education Today* **27**, 481–490.

Stuart, C.C. (2006) *Assessment, Supervision and Support in Clinical Practice – A Guide for Nurses, Midwives and Other Health Professionals*. Edinburgh: Churchill Livingstone Elsevier.

Watson, R., Stimpson, A., Topping, A. & Porock, D. (2002) 'Clinical competence assessment in nursing: a systematic review of the literature', *Journal of Advanced Nursing* **39**(5), 421–431.

WHO (2005) *Second International Consultation on WHO Guidelines in Hand Hygiene in Healthcare*. Implementation Strategies: Geneva.

Recommended reading

Baillie, L. (ed.) (2005) *Developing Practical Nursing Skills*. London: Hodder.

Brooker, C. & Waugh, A. (2007) *Foundations of Nursing Practice: Fundamentals of Holistic Care*. Edinburgh: Mosby Elsevier.

Dougherty, L. & Lister, S. (2008) *The Royal Marsden Hospital Manual of Clinical Nursing Procedures* (Royal Marsden NHS Trust). Oxford: Wiley-Blackwell.

Dougherty, L. & Lister, S. (2008) *The Royal Marsden Hospital Manual of Clinical Nursing Procedures* (student edition). Oxford: Wiley-Blackwell.

Entwistle, N. (2008) 'Teaching and learning research in Higher Education', review prepared for an international symposium, Guelph, Ontario, 25–26 April 2008.

Glasper, E. & Richardson, J. (eds) (2006) *A Textbook of Children's and Young People's Nursing*. London: Churchill Livingstone.

Henderson, C. & Macdonald, S. (eds) (2004) *Maye's Midwifery. A Textbook for Midwives* (13th edn). London: Bailliere Tindall.

Hinchliff, S., Norman, S. & Schober, J. (2008) *Nursing Practice and Health Care* (5th edn). London: Hodder Arnold.

Hughes, J. & Lyte, G. (2009) *Developing Nursing Practice with Children and Young People*. Chichester: Wiley-Blackwell.

Jones, A., Pegram, A. & Fordham-Clarke, A. (2009) 'Developing and examining an Objective Structured Clinical Examination'. *Nurse Education Today*. In press.

Maslin-Prothero, S. (ed.) (2005) *Baillière's Study Skills for Nurses and Midwives* (3rd edn). Edinburgh: Bailliere Tindall.

McCabe, C. & Timmins, F. (2006) *Communication Skills for Nursing Practice*. Basingstoke: Palgrave Macmillan.

Morrison, P. & Burnard, P. (1997) *Caring and Communicating: The Interpersonal Relationship in Nursing* (2nd edn). Basingstoke: Macmillan Education.

O'Carroll, M. & Park, A. (2007) *Essential Mental Health Nursing Skills*. Edinburgh: Mosby Elsevier.

Ross, M., Carroll, G., Knight, J., Chamberlain, M., Fothergill-Bourbonnais, F. & Linton, J. (1988) 'Using the OSCE to measure clinical skills performance in nursing', *Journal of Advanced Nursing* **13**, 45-56.

Wondrak, R.F. (1998) *Interpersonal Skills for Nurses and Health Care Professionals*. Oxford: Blackwell Science.

Useful website

CETL: Centre for Excellence in Teaching and Learning. Clinical & Communication Skills. www.cetl.org.uk/index.php

Index